High-Yield Immunology

SECOND EDITION

High-Yield Immunology

SECOND EDITION

Arthur G. Johnson, Ph.D.
Professor Emeritus
Department of Medical Microbiology and Immunology
University of Minnesota, Duluth, MN

Benjamin L. Clarke, Ph.D.
Associate Professor
Department of Medical Microbiology and Immunology
University of Minnesota Medical School, Duluth, MN

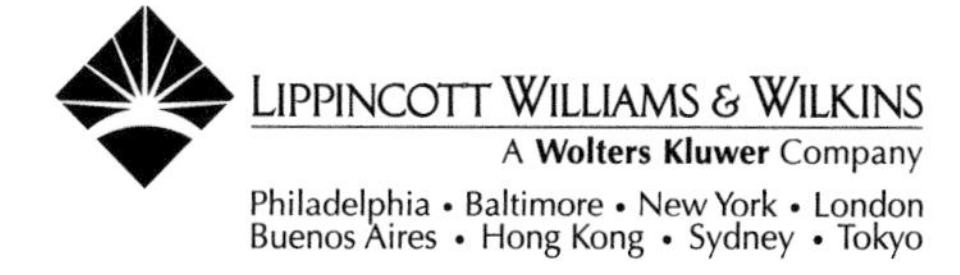

Acquisitions Editor: Betty Sun
Development Editor: Kathleen H. Scogna
Marketing Manager: Joe Schott
Production Editor: Jennifer D. Glazer
Designer: Doug Smock
Compositor: Circle Graphics, Inc.
Printer: Courier-Kendallville

351 West Camden Street
Baltimore, MD 21201

530 Walnut Street
Philadelphia, PA 19106

Printed in the United States of America

First Edition, 1999
Second Edition, 2005

Library of Congress Cataloging-in-Publication Data

Johnson, Arthur G.
High-yield immunology / Arthur G. Johnson, Benjamin L. Clarke.—2nd ed.
p. ; cm.
ISBN 0-7817-7469-1
1. Immunology—Outlines, syllabi, etc. I. Clarke, Benjamin L. II. Title.
[DNLM: 1. Immunity—Outlines 2. Hypersensitivity—Outlines. 3. Immunologic Factors—Outlines 4. Immunotherapy—Outlines. QW 18.2 J66h 2005]
QR182.55.J64 2005
616.07'9—dc22
2005047229

To purchase additional copies of this book, call our customer service department at (800) 638-3030 or fax orders to (301) 824-7390. International customers should call (301) 714-2324.

Visit Lippincott Williams & Wilkins on the Internet: http://www.LWW.com. Lippincott Williams & Wilkins customer service representatives are available from 8:30 am to 6:00 pm, EST.

06 07 08 09
2 3 4 5 6 7 8 9 10

Dedication

This edition of *High-Yield Immunology* is dedicated to our many students and colleagues, who have been a constant source of intellectual stimulation over the years.

Preface

High-Yield Immunology, 2nd edition, is a compendium of the knowledge considered necessary by the National Board of Medical Examiners (NBME) to achieve competence in immunology for the United States Medical Licensing Examination (USMLE). Immunology is a science that pervades most medical disciplines; this volume spans the breadth of the discipline and includes basic science, as well as clinical, information. We based our selection of what subject areas to include on the experience we have gleaned from years of teaching medical and graduate students. Topics, which include the following, are presented in a concise, "narrative outline" format:

- Development and function of the organs and cells involved in the immune response
- Properties of antigens and antibodies and the way they interact with each other
- Synthesis, genetic control, and regulation of antibody
- Cell-mediated immunity (CMI) and inflammation
- Immunologic disorders, including hypersensitivity disorders, immunodeficiency disorders, and autoimmune diseases
- The role of the immune system in transplantation and cancer
- Currently available vaccines and recommended immunization schedules
- Addition of three new chapters:
  - Innate Immunity
  - Signal Transduction in Immune Cells
  - Study questions and answers

Numerous tables and illustrations round out the presentation by summarizing information and clarifying difficult concepts.

This book is not meant to replace the many excellent textbooks of immunology. Rather, it is our hope that the concise presentation of information in *High-Yield Immunology* will assist the reader in the quick recall of the facts considered essential for understanding this exciting and rapidly changing science.

Acknowledgments

We would like to thank Tenille Sands, Managing Editor, for her professionalism and organization, which kept the project moving smoothly. In addition, we would like to thank Carmen DiBartolomeo and Beach Studios, who created the art program for the book. Last but not least, we would like to thank many of our colleagues, whose diligent research over the years has provided much of the current medical insight into the concepts and disorders described herein.

Art Johnson
Ben Clarke

Contents

Chapter **1**

Overview

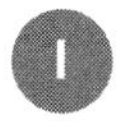

SYNOPSIS. The immune system is a complex system composed of several types of sessile and mobile cells that interact in lymphoid tissue dispersed throughout the body. This system is stimulated by the introduction of foreign material (**antigen**) into the host; its function is the elimination of this material.

A. Organs involved:
  1. **Central lymphoid organs** (where immunocompetent cells are developed)
     a. Thymus
     b. Bone marrow
  2. **Peripheral lymphoid organs** (where immunocompetency is expressed)
     a. Spleen
     b. Lymph nodes
     c. Tonsils
     d. Intestinal Peyer's patches
     e. Mucosa

B. Cells involved:
  1. **Antigen-presenting cells (APCs), thymus-derived (T) cells,** and **bone marrow–derived (B) cells** interact in the organs to produce two types of acquired immunity.
     a. **Humoral immunity (HI)** is mediated by proteins called **antibodies,** which neutralize microorganisms and toxins and remove antigens in the body fluids by **amplifying phagocytosis or lysis.**
     b. **Cellular (cell-mediated) immunity (CMI)** is mediated by **T cytotoxic (TC) cells, natural killer (NK) cells, polymorphonuclear (PMN) cells,** and **macrophages** and is responsible for **eradicating microorganisms residing within body cells,** as well as **killing aberrant host cells.**

II **CONCERNS IN MEDICINE** include:

A. The immune system's role in protection against infectious diseases and cancer
B. Immune-mediated complications of organ transplantation
C. The immune system's role in allergic disorders
D. The immune system's role in autoimmune disorders
E. The development of specific, sensitive assays for the diagnosis of disease

III **HOST-PARASITE EQUILIBRIUM** is largely in favor of the host. Whether the host or parasite prevails depends on whether the parasite's pathogenicity can overcome the host's immunity.

A. Attributes of the parasite
  1. **Communicability:** the transfer of microorganisms between individuals or via vectors
  2. **Penetrability:** the ability of the microorganism to gain access into the host

3. **Invasiveness:** the ability of the microorganism to enter the tissues
4. **Toxigenicity:** the ability of the microorganism to inflict damage on the host

B. Attributes of the host

1. **Innate (native) immunity is nonspecific** and encompasses factors present in an individual independent of antigenic stimulus (e.g., **skin, mucous membranes, sebaceous secretions, pinocytosis, phagocytosis**). (See Chapter 3)
2. **Acquired immunity (HI and CMI)**
   a. **Actively acquired** by:
      (1) Infection
      (2) Vaccination
   b. **Passively acquired** by:
      (1) Placental transfer of antibody
      (2) Injection of specific antibody or cells

DEVELOPMENT OF THE ACQUIRED IMMUNE SYSTEM

A. Multipotential stem cells originate in the **fetal liver and bone marrow.**

1. **T cells.** When stem cells migrate to the fetal thymus, they acquire the phenotypic characteristics of T cells under the influence of thymic hormones (Figure 1.1).
   a. **Clusters of differentiation (CD).** These phenotypic markers appear on the T cell membrane as proteins at different stages of differentiation in the thymus and periphery.
      (1) **CD2 and CD3** are major markers that appear in the thymus and are retained on all *peripheral* T cells.
      (2) **CD4** defines a **T helper cell (Th) subset**, which differentiates in the periphery into **Th0, Th1,** and **Th2 cells** based on differences in the molecules they secrete (known as **cytokines**).
         (a) **Th1 cells** secrete mainly **interleukin-2 (IL-2), interferon-γ (IFN-γ),** and **tumor necrosis factor-α** (TNF-α).
         (b) **Th2 cells secrete** mainly **IL-4, IL-5, IL-6, IL-10,** and **IL-13.**
      (3) **CD8** defines a **T cytotoxic–suppressor cell (Tc or Ts) subset**, active in CMI.
   b. **The T cell antigenic receptor (TCR)** is **epitope specific** and exists on the T cell membrane as two types, designated **α:βTCR** and **γ:δTCR.**
   c. Approximately 1%–2% of T cells leave the thymus and enter the peripheral tissues; the remaining T cells die in **apoptosis**, characterized by condensation and fragmentation of nuclei and membrane blebbing.
   d. A T cell–dependent **homing area** exists periarteriolarly in the spleen, in the paracortical and deep cortical regions in the lymph nodes, and in the gastrointestinal-associated and bronchus-associated tissues.
2. **B cells**
   a. If stem cells remain in the bone marrow, they acquire the phenotypic CD markers characteristic of the stages of **B cell differentiation** (Figure 1.2).
   b. A **membrane-bound, epitope-specific, antigenic receptor** that is a **monomeric immunoglobulin M (IgM) antibody** distinguishes the B cell antigenic receptor from that of the T cell.
   c. **B cell homing areas** exist primarily in the splenic follicles and red pulp, the lymph nodes, and mucosal-associated tissues.

B. Partial maturation of T cells in the thymus and B cells in the bone marrow in utero is followed by migration to and seeding of the peripheral lymphoid tissues. After birth, the T and B cells differentiate further in peripheral lymphoid tissue and gain immunocompetency under antigenic stimulus.

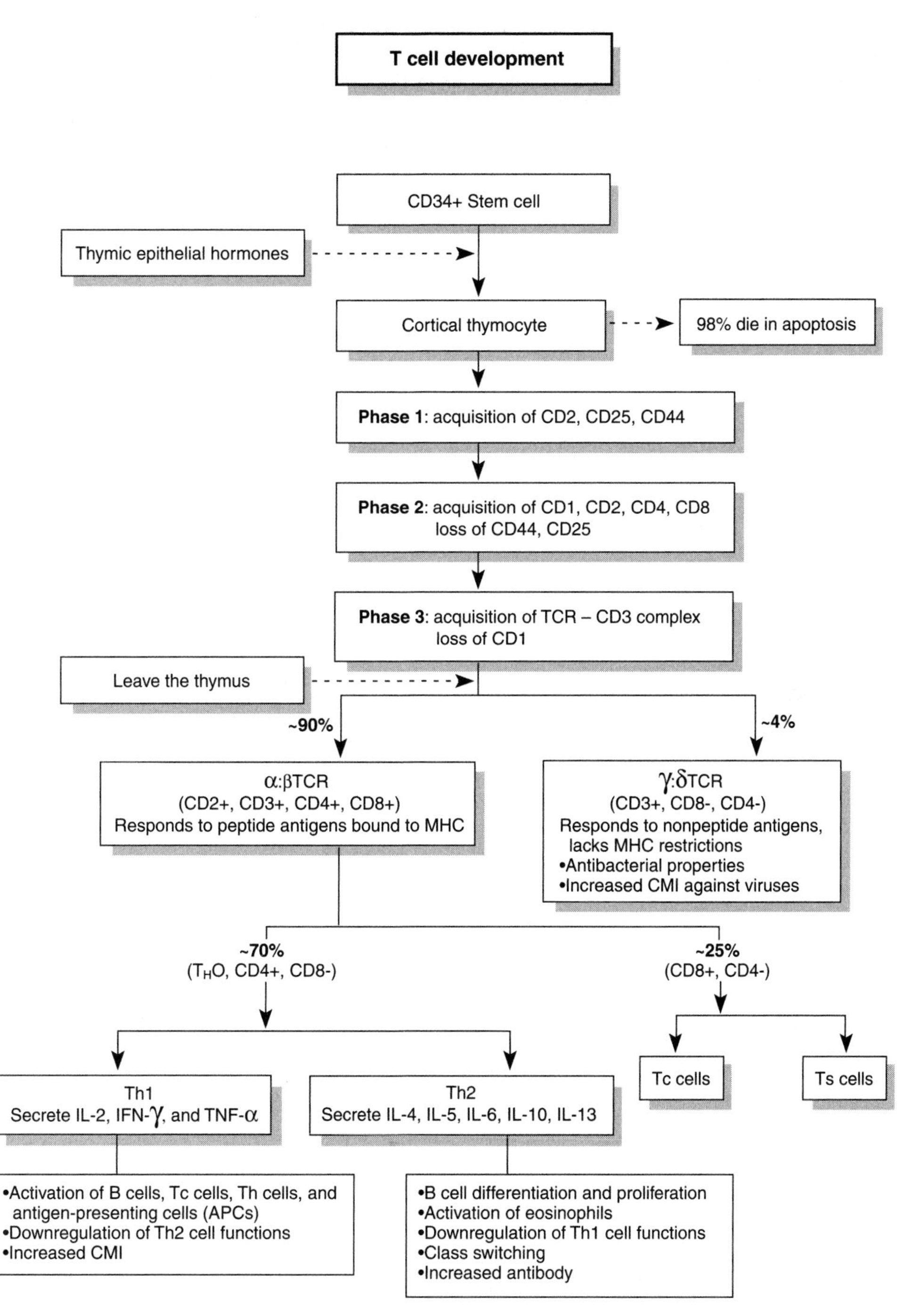

● **Figure 1.1** T cell development. Stem cells from bone marrow bearing a CD34 marker migrate to the fetal thymus, where they become cortical thymocytes under the influence of epithelial hormones. Most of the cortical thymocytes die; the surviving 1%–2% pass through three phases of development, during which they acquire and lose specific membrane markers [clusters of differentiation *(CD)*]. During the final phase, which takes place in the medulla, the thymocytes acquire the T cell antigenic receptor *(TCR)* and the CD3 signaling complex, and they lose the CD1 marker and leave the thymus. The T cells can have one of two types of TCR (α:βTCR or γ:δTCR); the types are differentiated according to the amino acids in the two peptide chains that form the receptor. The α:βTCR T cells respond to peptide antigens bound to the major histocompatibility complex *(MHC)*, while the γ:δTCR T cells respond to nonpeptide antigens. There are two populations of α:βTCR T cells, Th1 cells and Th2 cells. These cells secrete different cytokines and therefore have different functions. *CMI* = cell-mediated immunity; *IL* = interleukin; *IFN* = interferon; *Tc* = cytotoxic T (cell); *Th* = T helper (cell); *Ts* = T suppressor (cell).

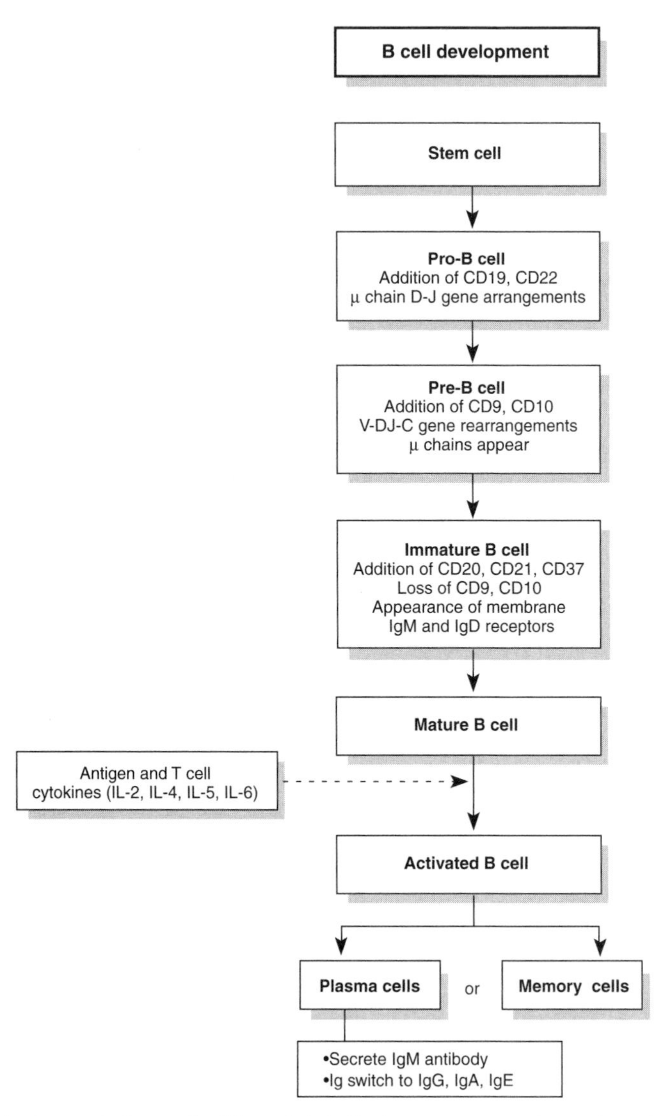

● **Figure 1.2** B cell development. Stem cells differentiate in the bone marrow and pass through several stages of development before becoming mature B cells. Random selection by each B cell from a variety of germ line genes results in a large number of possible structures for the epitope-binding regions of the immunoglobulins. At the pro-B cell stage, a joining *(J)* region gene links with a diversity *(D)* segment gene. At the pre-B cell stage, the DJ complex links with a variable *(V)* region gene, and then the VDJ complex links to the μ constant *(C)* region gene (see Chapter 5). At the immature B cell stage, the appearance of membrane IgM and IgD receptors defines B cell clones. Activation of the mature B cells by antigen and T cell cytokines leads to differentiation and division of the B cells and synthesis of antibody. *CD* = cluster of differentiation.

V **CLONAL SELECTION THEORY.** Expression of acquired immunity is governed conceptually by the clonal selection theory: the total population of T cells as well as the total population of B cells in the body is made up of millions of individual clones of cells, each clone defined by the occurrence of a **specific receptor for a particular antigen epitope.** On entry, antigen is modified by APCs and selects T cells, B cells, or both possessing the membrane-bound receptor specific for its epitope. Cytokine-induced differentiation and expansion of only that clone follows through division. Thus, only T and B cell clones specific for the particular organism responsible for the patient's disease increase to adequate numbers and function to eradicate the pathogen.

Chapter 2
Antigens

I DEFINITIONS

A. Antigen is a foreign substance that induces antibody and/or CMI after binding to its specific antigenic receptor on T and B cell clones.

B. Epitope (antigenic determinant, ligand). An epitope is the short sequence of amino acids or sugars in an antigen molecule that combines with a hypervariable reactive site on the antibody molecule. The sequence is usually repeated several times, and the number of repeats is referred to as the **valence.**

C. Hapten. A hapten is a portion of an antigen molecule that contains the epitope. This area reacts specifically with its antibody but is incapable of inducing antibody synthesis without a carrier molecule.

D. Superantigen. Certain retroviral proteins and bacterial toxins (e.g., staphylococcal enterotoxins, toxic shock syndrome toxin 1) can link multiple T cells—at the T cell receptor (TCR) Vβ regions—to the major histocompatibility complex (MHC, class II) of antigen-presenting cells (APCs). Because this linking occurs at regions independent of the specific peptide-binding sites, many T cell clones and APCs are activated, secreting excessive amounts of cytokines (e.g., IL-2, IL-1), potentially resulting in toxic shock syndrome.

E. Thymus-independent antigens activate B cells without T helper cell (Th) involvement. Most thymus-independent antigens possess multiple branched polysaccharide repeating units (e.g., lipopolysaccharides from Gram-negative bacteria) and activate B cells polyclonally, without regard to B cell specificity (B cell mitogens).

II FACTORS DETERMINING ANTIGENICITY.

Antigens are usually protein or polysaccharide; lipids are poorly antigenic. Factors that determine antigenicity include:

A. Degree of "foreignness" and host background

B. Size, shape, chemical composition of the antigen, and amount, route, and frequency of exposure

III EXAMPLES OF ANTIGENS

A. Microorganisms

1. Frequently, **bacterial antigens** can be components of virulence of the organism. Therefore, **attenuated or killed vaccines** should retain the antigens that are important for virulence.
2. **Antigenic mosaics** are the basis for **serologic classification.**
    a. **Streptococcal antigens** are exemplified by group-specific carbohydrates, type-specific M proteins, streptolysin O, erythrogenic toxins, and multiple enzymes.
    b. ***Salmonella* antigens** are exemplified by O antigen (lipopolysaccharide), H (flagellar) antigen, virulence (Vi) antigen, pili, and several exotoxins.

(1) Terminal sugars with varying optical isomerism determine different species.

(2) Cross-reactions can occur with closely related epitopes.

c. **Human immunodeficiency virus (HIV) antigens** are exemplified by glycoproteins (e.g., gp160, gp120, gp41) and enzymes (e.g., reverse transcriptase). The numerical designation of the glycoproteins refers to the molecular weight.

B. Human tissue antigens

1. Blood-group antigens (see Table 10.2).
2. Organ-specific antigens (see Chapter 12).
3. Individual-specific leukocytic antigens (e.g., human leukocyte antigens [HLA]) (see Tables 5.1 and 5.2).

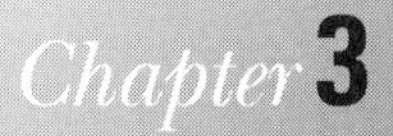

Chapter 3 Innate Immunity

I FUNDAMENTAL CHARACTERISTICS

A. **Initial rapid recognition system** for detecting pathogens
B. Genetically programmed without host adaptation; nonspecific
C. Physical barriers and phagocytic cells **restrain** infectious agents
D. Sentinel cells identify pathogens and **recruit** other cells using cytokines
E. Microorganisms are processed and peptide fragments presented to T cells, thus initiating and coordinating the acquired response
F. The acute phase response is activated and provides additional bloodborne components to augment or regulate innate immune responses

II DEFENSIVE MECHANISMS

A. Barriers
  1. Skin blocks pathogen entry
  2. Mucous membranes form a fluid barrier to flush away pathogen
B. Entrapment (clotting, sebaceous secretions)
C. Secreted enzymes are
  1. Lysozyme, released into lachrymal and saliva secretions
  2. Perforins and granzymes are released to initiate apoptosis killing
D. Anti-microbial peptides
  1. Defensins are
    a. A small group of cationic peptides (nine genes) that damage bacterial membranes
    b. Found in cytoplasmic granules of phagocytic and secretory cells
    c. A major component of the azurophil granules in neutrophils
    d. Released into the phagocytic vacuole
  2. Surfactants A and D are
    a. Lung secretions that bath epithelial linings
    b. Capable of coating the surfaces of pathogens to facilitate phagocytosis by macrophages
  3. Cathelicidins are
    a. A large family of antimicrobial peptides
    b. Stored in secretory granules in a precursor form
    c. Released from the cell and activated by extracellular protease activity
    d. Able to make bacterial membranes permeable
E. Alternate complement pathway (see Figure 6.4)
  1. Independent of antibody or mannan-binding lectin pathways
  2. Spontaneously hydrolyzes C3 in the plasma and forms a multiprotein complex, C3 convertase, that can randomly bind to any pathogen or host membrane surface possessing thioester linkages
  3. Properdin (factor P) binds to bacterial surfaces and augments C3 convertase activity

4. Host cells express surface regulatory proteins that suppress C3 convertase to prevent inadvertent complement action
5. Complement pathways lead to opsonization or lysis of pathogen

F. Phagocytosis

1. Neutrophils are
   a. Polymorphonuclear leukocytes (PMN)
   b. The earliest and most abundant respondent cell to pathogen invasion
   c. An important protective cell since hereditary deficiencies are fatal because of overwhelming bacterial infections
2. Macrophages are
   a. Derived from their monocytic precursor following stimulation by granulocyte-macrophage–colony stimulating factor (GM-CSF)
   b. Highly phagocytic, utilizing their Fc receptor or complement receptors to capture antibody or complement associated pathogens
   c. Capable of killing intracellular pathogens with super-oxygen radicals and lysosome enzymatic digestion
3. Dendritic cells (see Figure 3.1)
   a. Present in two forms
      (1) When **immature**, they are highly phagocytic, itinerate cells (iDC) expressing low MHC levels that capture and process pathogens into antigenic fragments
      (2) Exposure to pathogen molecules activates toll-like receptors (TLR) to stimulate differentiation into **mature** dendritic cells (mDC)
      (3) When **mature**, they are sessile, non-phagocytic and express abundant MHC in secondary lymphoid organs. This results in a **display of antigenic peptides to naïve T-cells.**

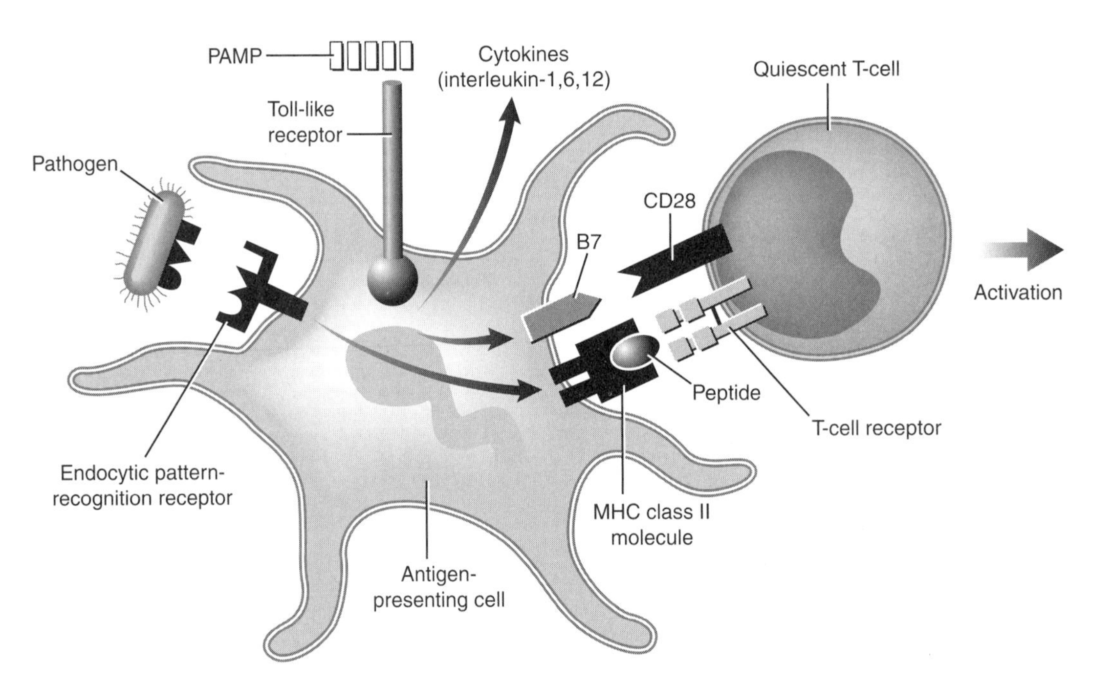

● **Figure 3.1** Dendritic cells activate naïve T cells. (Modified with permission from Medzhitov R, Janeway C Jr. Innate immunity. N Engl J Med 2000; 343(5):342.) iDC cells differentiate into mDC when PAMPs bind to Toll-like receptors. Antigen displayed on MHC class II molecules are presented to specific T cells where recognition is defined by the TCR. Further selection is made by the co-receptor (e.g., CD4, not shown) and co-stimulatory molecules (e.g., B7).

b. Initially, mDC dock to T cells via a peptide MHC to TCR linkage. The resulting T cell response is regulated by either CD4 or CD8 linkage to the MHC. Activation of T cells requires B7 or CD86 (on DC) linkage to CD28 (on T cell). Failure of the B7-CD28 linkage commits the T cell to a perpetual tolerant state called **anergy**.

G. Natural killer (NK) cells are (see Figure 3.2)

1. Lymphoid derived, granular secretory cells.

2. Cells expressing both Fc receptors and CD56 and producing interferon-γ.

3. Deficient in expressing antigen-specific membrane receptors or memory, and are not MHC restricted.

4. Capable of identifying cells expressing **low levels of MHC class I** (e.g., virus-infected cells or those transformed into cancer) and are indiscriminate in binding to all host cells.

MHC class I on normal cells is recognized by killer inhibitory receptors (KIRs) or by lectinlike CD94:NKG2 heterodimers on NK cells, which inhibit signals from activating receptors

NK cell does not kill the normal cell

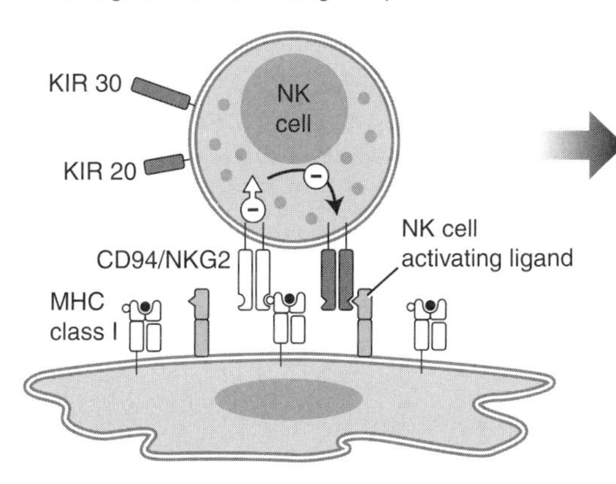

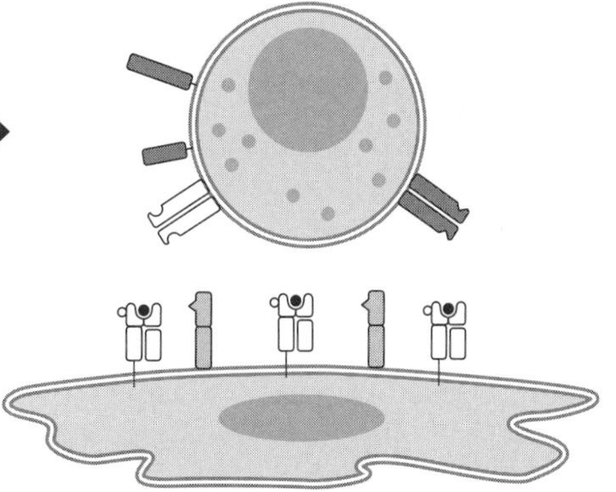

"Altered" or absent MHC class I cannot stimulate a negative signal. NK cell is triggered by signals from activating receptors

Activated NK cell releases granule contents, inducing apoptosis in target cell

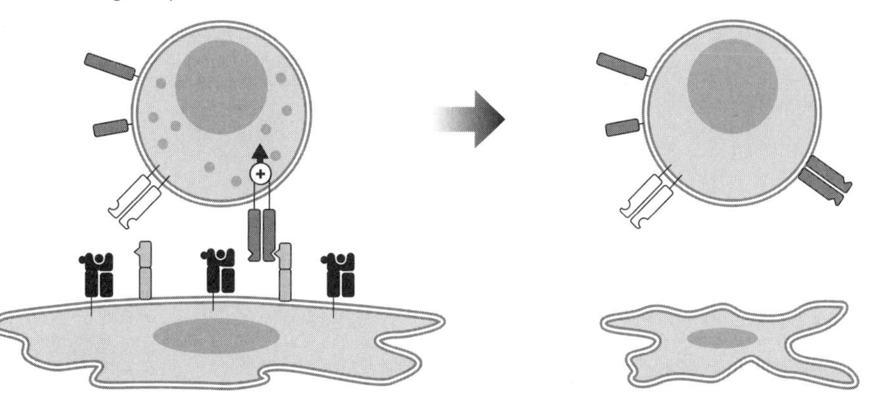

● **Figure 3.2** Recognition of infected cells by NK cells. (Modified with permission from Janeway CA, Travers P, Walport M, Shlomchik MJ: Immunobiology, 5th ed. NY, Garland Publishing, 2001, p 84.) Host cells exposed to IFN-α and INF-β are induced to express MHC class I molecules; however, some infected cells do not express MHC class I that would reveal the presence of pathogen. NK cells survey host cells for deficient MHC class I expression to target infected cells for killing.

5. Capable of initiating a killing response to any docked cells using a killer-activating receptor (KAR). Apoptosis is induced in the target cell using perforins and granzymes.
6. Capable of halting inadvertent **host** cell death by recognizing the presence of MHC complexes on the target cell through killer inhibitory receptors (KIR).

III ACUTE PHASE RESPONSE (APR)

A. Responds rapidly to tissue damage causing the release of cytokines from macrophages.
B. The cytokines IL-1, IL-6, and TNF-α stimulate an increase in select serum proteins originating predominately from the liver.
C. APR proteins are used to augment immune responses (complement), regulate the extent of response (protease inhibitors, e.g., α1-antitrypsin), or stimulate additional responses (α_2-macroglobulin).

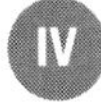

IV PATHOGEN RECOGNITION SYSTEMS

A. Antigen-presenting cells (APC).

Cell Type	Function	MHC Class II Expression	Outcome to Immune Challenge
Macrophage	a) Sentinel—detects pathogen via receptor for f-met-peptides of bacterial origin b) Restricts invasion c) Recruits other immunocytes d) Promotes cell-mediated response e) Phagocytosis is directed by antibody and complement	Medium	a) Pathogen is engulfed and destroyed, and fragment released for iDC capture b) Cytokine production (IL-1, IL-6, TNF-α) c) CMI is recruited and activated
B-cell lymphocyte	Uptake of soluble material via surface immunoglobulin	Medium	a) To produce antibody b) Rapid response to a secondary challenge (memory cell effect)
Immature dendritic cell (iDC)	a) Roams tissues as a sentinel b) Phagocytosis gathers soluble material	Low	Processing pathogens into fragments for MHC display
Mature dendritic cell (mDC)	Abundant membrane display of antigen	Very High	a) Antigen display for presentation to naïve T cells b) TLR activation induces B7 expression to permit T cell activation c) Secretes IL-12, which induces NK and T_h1 CMI

B. Host receptors for unique pathogen structures
1. Characteristics
   a. Genetically predetermined recognition receptors for pathogens on host cell, called pattern-recognition receptors (PAR), examples are **TLR** and **endocytosis receptors.**
   b. These recognize a few highly conserved structures expressed in a large group of microorganisms, but not humans. These structures are referred to as **pathogen-associated molecular patterns** (PAMPs).
2. PAMPs

a. Pathogen-specific molecules, which are essential for pathogen survival.
b. Invariant, a trait shared by an entire class of pathogens.
c. Examples: lipopolysaccharide, peptidoglycan, lipoteichoic acid, mannans, bacterial DNA, double-strand RNA, glucans.

C. Major histocompatibility complex (MHC)—refer to Chapters 5 and 13

D. Killer-activating receptor (KAR) (see Figure 3.2)

1. Characteristics
a. Found on NK cells
b. Binds to host cells by recognizing ubiquitous surface molecule
c. Screens for MHC class I expression
d. Initiates NK killing activity in cells with **diminished MHC class I** content by inducing apoptosis in the target cell

2. Regulated by MHC class I expression
a. To halt killing action of KAR, a KIR binds to MHC class I
b. If KIR is not bound, the NK cell to proceed with killing
c. Viral infection and cancer cells commonly have reduced MHC class I expression, thus favoring NK killing response

E. Coordination of cell-mediated immune response driven by innate immunity

1. Characteristics
a. Innate immunity involves integrating signals derived from MHC class II, TLR, and docking of co-receptor B7 on mDC.
b. Triggering of these three signals results in the release of IL-12 from APC.
c. Complete signaling stimulates T cell proliferation and differentiation; incomplete signaling forces the T cell to enter anergy.

2. Function
a. MHC class I expression stimulates cytotoxic immune responses.
b. MHC class II expression stimulates humoral immune responses.
c. Activation of TLR signals the presence of a pathogen and determines if a cell-mediated immune response is required.

F. Coordination of innate immune responses driven by acquired immunity (see Figure 3.3)

1. Characteristics
a. Receptors on innate immune cells are used to bind recognition molecules.
(1) Complement receptors found on macrophages bind antigen-antibody-complement complexes.
(2) Fc receptors found on macrophages and eosinophils bind antibodies.
b. Large pools of non-specific, latent effector cells are quickly transformed into specific effector cells by binding antigen-antibody or antigen-antibody complement complexes or by non-specific macrophage stimulants such as Gram-negative bacterial lipopolysaccharides.

2. Function
a. Integration of HI and CMI with innate immunity
b. Associated with host defenses to parasites and allergic responses
c. Opsonization

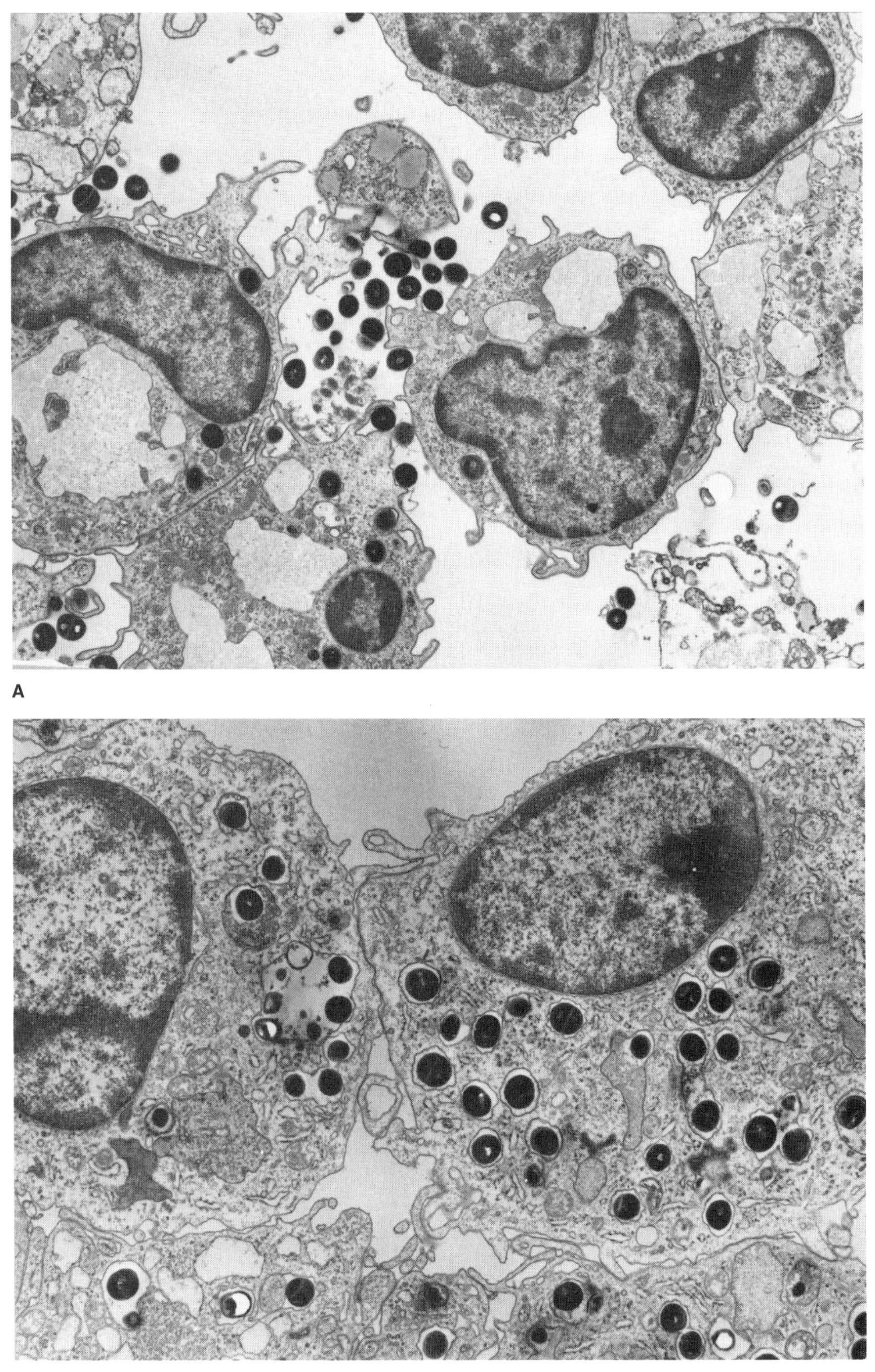

● **Figure 3.3** Amplification of innate immunity by acquired immunity. *(A)* Normal murine macrophages exposed to *Staphylococcus aureus* for 5 minutes immediately before fixation. Note only a few bacterial cells are phagocytized. *(B)* Addition of anti-S. aureus antibody results in phagocytosis of most of the bacterial cells.

Chapter **4**

Antibodies

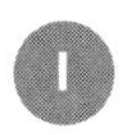

GENERAL PROPERTIES

A. Definition. Antibodies are mucoproteins that are found mainly in the γ-globulin fraction of serum on electrophoresis. These mucoproteins are called **immunoglobulins (Ig).**

B. Heterogeneity

1. **Five classes.** When injected into animals, human immunoglobulin, being foreign, becomes antigenic. The resulting antihuman immunoglobulin antibodies are grouped into five classes: **IgG, IgA, IgM, IgE, and IgD.**
2. **Structure.** The basic structural unit for each class is a four-chain protein with two heavy (H) and two light (L) chain polypeptides linked by disulphide bonds (Figure 4.1).
   a. **Amino acid sequences**
      (1) **H chains.** A specific, short amino acid sequence on the H chains differentiates the classes (i.e., IgG, IgA, IgM, IgE, IgD). These H-chain differences are called **isotypes** and are designated by the Greek letters **gamma (γ), alpha (α), mu (μ), epsilon (ε),** and **delta (δ),** respectively. Isotypes are genetic variations that all normal humans possess.
      (2) **L chains**
         (a) All five classes have an amino acid sequence in common on the L chains. Thus, they can be classified together as immunoglobulins.
         (b) In addition, two L-chain isotypes, designated **kappa (κ)** and **lambda (λ),** exist for all five classes.
   b. **Amino acid composition.** Both H and L chains are divided into **constant region domains** (designated CH and CL) and **variable region domains** (designated VH and VL).
      (1) **Constant region domains.** The amino acid sequence in the constant regions of both the H and L chains is similar for all antibody molecules within each class.
      (2) **Variable region domains.** The amino acid sequence of the variable regions on both H and L chains varies with the epitope toward which the particular antibody is directed.
         (a) Amino acids that show marked differences between antibodies of different specificities form the **hypervariable region** within each variable region.
         (b) The hypervariable regions of both the H and L chains associate to form the **epitope-binding region,** of which there are two, known as the antibody **idiotype.**
      (3) A **hinge region** also exists between the CH_1 and CH_2 domains, permitting flexibility in the movement of the two antigen-binding sites.

C. Monoclonal antibodies. Most antigenic preparations give rise to a mixture of antibodies. However, antibodies of a single specificity are highly desirable for many

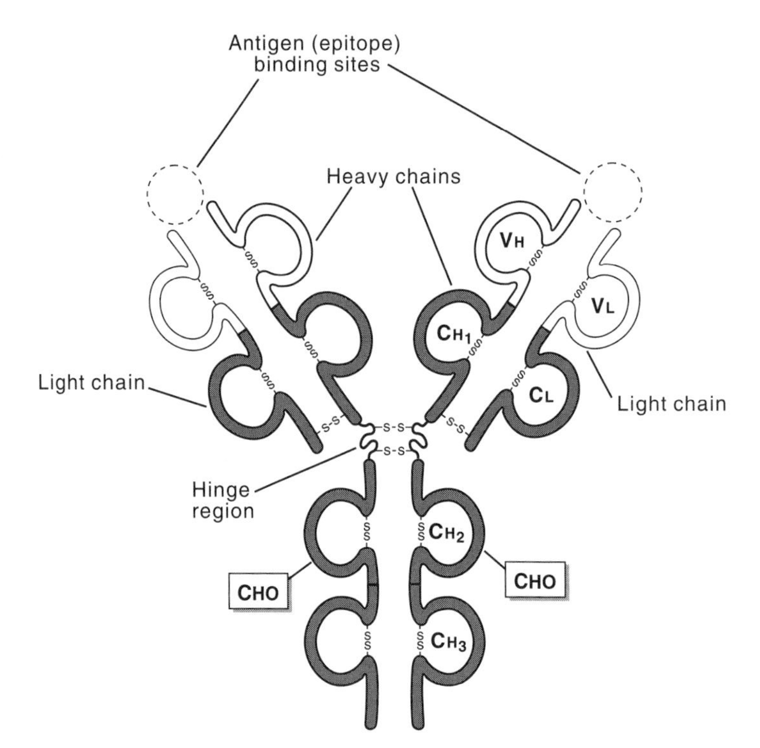

● **Figure 4.1** The basic four-peptide structure of immunoglobulins is illustrated by this IgG pattern. Three heavy chain constant region domains (CH_1, CH_2, CH_3) and one light chain constant domain (C_L) are shown in *black*. The variable region of both the light and heavy chains (V_L and V_H, respectively; in *white*) associate to form the specific epitope-binding site. Several of the most critical disulfide bonds are shown (*—ss—*). *CHO* indicates where the carbohydrate is attached. (Redrawn with permission from Eisen HN: *General Immunology*. Philadelphia, Lippincott-Raven, 1990, p 48.)

purposes, including specific diagnostic tests and immunotherapy. Monoclonal antibodies can be made routinely.

1. Splenic B cells from an immunized animal are fused with malignant (immortal) plasma cells, forming a **hybridoma.**
2. The B cell hybridoma secreting the desired antibody can be isolated from the others by reactivity with the antigen of concern, cloned and expanded in tissue culture, resulting in large amounts of antibody of a single specificity.

D. Humanized antibodies

1. Immunotherapeutic regimens are being developed using monoclonal mouse–human chimeric antibodies to human cancer-specific antigens to destroy certain cancer cells (e.g., B cell lymphomas).
2. Such antibodies are constructed by combining the murine gene for the variable region (Fab) of the anti-cancer antibody (which contributes the desired specificity), together with the human gene for the constant region (Fc) of the desired human isotype (thus diminishing the "foreignness" of the antibody).
3. Infusion of the antibody into patients causes complement mediated lysis of the cancer cell.

E. Immunotoxins

1. Monoclonal antibodies can also be constructed using the Fab domain from a murine antibody against a cancer-specific antigen with the mouse Fc domain removed and displaced by any number of different toxins.
2. Such antibodies bind specifically to the cancer cell antigen via the mouse Fab hypervariable region, thereby focusing the lethal toxin on only the designated target cell.

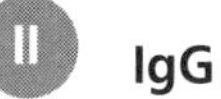

IgG

A. Structural properties (Table 4.1)

1. **Molecular weight.** IgG is composed of two L chains (each with a molecular weight of 22,000 d) and two H chains (each with a molecular weight of 53,000 d). The total molecular weight is 150,000 d.
2. The **structural designation** is ($\gamma_2\kappa_2$) or ($\gamma_2\lambda_2$), with the γ-marker indicating the IgG H-chain isotype and the κ- or λ-marker indicating the L-chain isotype.
3. **Four subclasses exist: γ_1, γ_2, γ_3, and γ_4.** These subclasses are differentiated by slight changes in the amino acid sequences on the λ H chain.
4. **Enzymatic cleavage (Figure 4.2)**
   a. **Papain** splits IgG into three fragments.
      (1) Two of these fragments (**Fab; fragment, antigen binding**) are similar, with each containing only one of the reactive sites for the epitope. Because Fab is monovalent, it can bind to but cannot enter into lattice formation and precipitate or agglutinate antigen.
      (2) A third fragment (**Fc; crystallizable**) activates complement, controls catabolism of IgG, fixes IgG to tissues or cells via an Fc receptor, and mediates placental transfer.
   b. **Pepsin** splits behind the disulphide bond joining the two H chains, permitting the two Fab fragments to remain joined. Consequently, this fragment is termed F(**ab′**)2.
      (1) Because F(ab′)2 is bivalent, it is capable of lattice formation and aggregation of antigens.
      (2) F(ab′)2 is removed more rapidly from the circulation than the intact IgG.
      (3) The Fc fragment is extensively degraded.

B. Functional properties (Table 4.2)

1. **Serum and half-life.** IgG has the highest serum concentration of all immunoglobulins (700–1500 mg%) and a serum half-life of 18–25 days.
2. **Functions**
   a. IgG adheres to cells that possess a receptor for the Fc fragment from IgG (Fcγ).

TABLE 4.1 STRUCTURAL PROPERTIES OF HUMAN IMMUNOGLOBULINS

Property	IgG	IgM	IgA	IgE	IgD
H-chain isotype	γ	μ	α	ϵ	δ
H-chain subclass	γ_1, γ_2, γ_3, γ_4	. . .	α_1, α_2	. . .	. . .
L-chain isotype	κ or λ	κ or λ	κ or λ	κ or λ	κ or λ
Associated chains	. . .	J chain	J chain, SP	. . .	. . .
Structural designation	$\gamma_2\kappa_2$ or $\gamma_2\lambda_2$	$(\mu_2\kappa_2)_5$ or $(\mu_2\lambda_2)_5$	**Serum:** $\alpha\kappa_2$ or $\alpha\gamma_2$ **Mucosa:** $(\alpha_2\kappa_2)_2$ J, SP or $(\alpha_2\gamma_2)_2$ J, SP	$\epsilon_2\kappa_2$ or $\epsilon_2\lambda_2$	$\delta_2\kappa_2$ or $\delta_2\lambda_2$
Percent carbohydrate	4	15	10	18	18
Molecular weight (daltons)	150,000	**Monomer:** 180,000 **Pentamer:** 950,000	**Monomer:** 160,000 **Dimer:** 318,000 **Dimer + SP:** 380,000	188,000	184,000

J = J chain; SP = secretory piece.

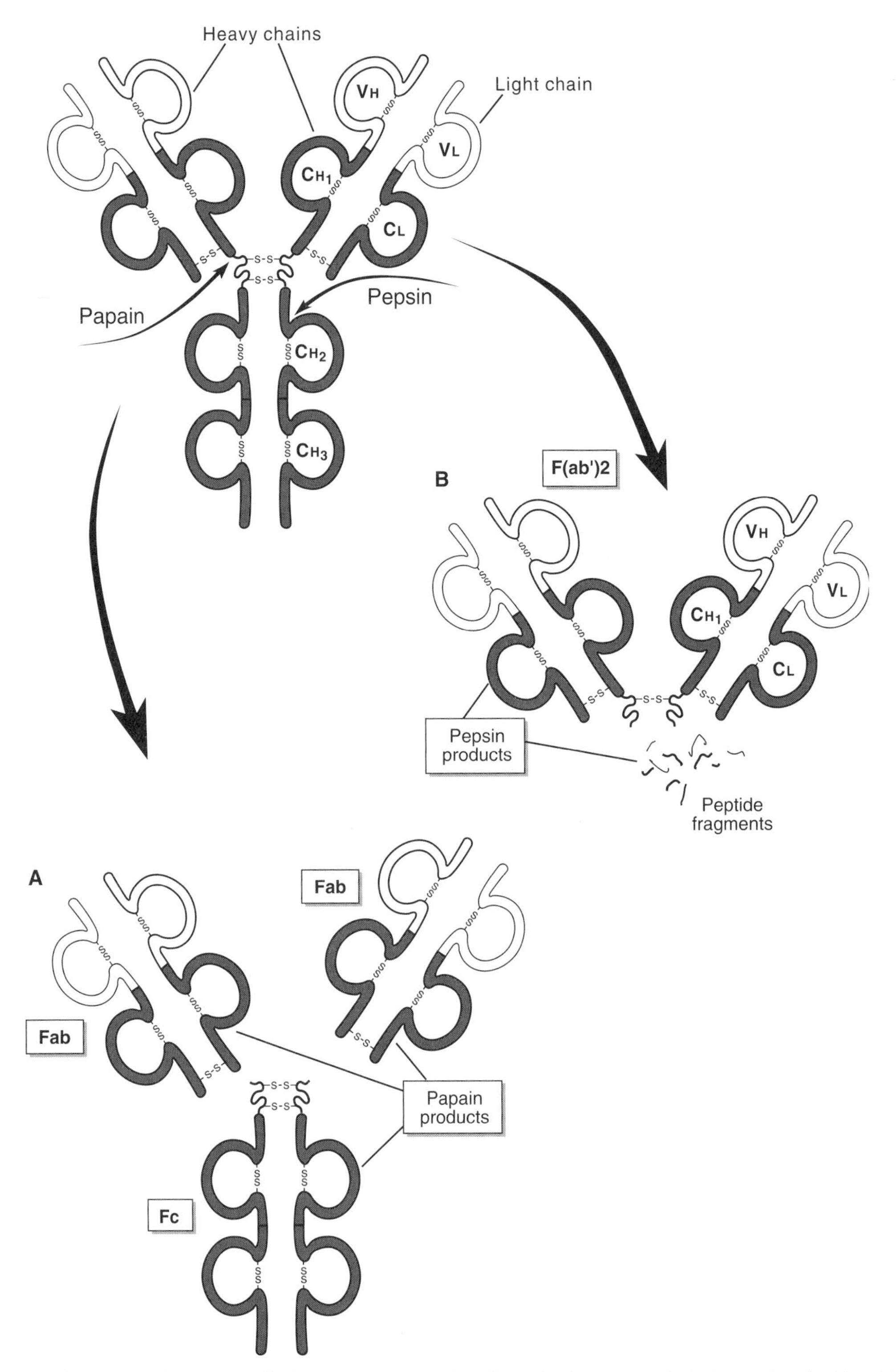

● **Figure 4.2** Enzymatic cleavage of IgG by pepsin and papain. (*A*) Papain cleavage results in two unlinked antigen binding (Fab) fragments with the disulphide bonds (*—ss—*) remaining with the crystallizable (Fc) fragment. Because the fragments are univalent, they cannot precipitate or agglutinate antigens. (*B*) Pepsin cleavage results in retention of the disulphide bonds with the two Fab fragments linked as F(ab')2. The Fc portion is degraded. CH_1, CH_2, CH_3 = heavy chain constant region domains; V_L, V_H = variable region of light and heavy chains, respectively. (Redrawn with permission from Abbas AK, Lichtman AH, Pober JS: *Cellular and Molecular Immunology,* 3rd ed. Philadelphia, WB Saunders, 1997, p 50.)

TABLE 4.2 FUNCTIONAL PROPERTIES OF HUMAN IMMUNOGLOBULINS

Property	IgG γ_1	IgG γ_2	IgG γ_3	IgG γ_4	IgM	IgA α_1	IgA α_2	IgE	IgD
Average serum concentration (mg%)	900	300	100	50	150	300	50	0.03	3
Serum half-life (days)	23	23	8	23	5	5	5	3	2.5
Activates complement	+	±	++	−	+++	−	−	−	−
Binds to Fc receptor	+	±	++	+	+	−	−	+	−
Crosses placenta	+	±	+	+	−	−	−	−	−

b. IgG fixes complement (i.e., a series of enzymes resulting in cell lysis).
c. IgG mediates placental passage of maternal antibody to the fetus.

III IgM

A. Structural properties (see Table 4.1)

1. **Form.** IgM exists in two structural forms.
   a. A **monomer** is synthesized by and retained on the membrane of B cells and is designated $\mu_2\kappa_2$ or $\mu_2\lambda_2$.
      (1) A monomer serves as the B cell receptor specific for a single antigenic epitope.
      (2) The hypervariable region of the monomer differs for each B cell clone.
   b. Secreted IgM exists as a **pentamer** (i.e., five monomeric IgM molecules joined together by a J chain; Figure 4.3). The IgM pentamer is designated $(\mu_2\kappa_2)_5$ or $(\mu_2\lambda_2)_5$.
      (1) The pentamer is secreted following antigen and cytokine activation of plasma cells, with the hypervariable regions on the pentamer the same as those on the membrane-bound monomeric receptor.
      (2) Of the 10 possible epitope-binding sites on the pentamer, five are of high affinity and five are of low affinity.
2. **Molecular weight.** IgM has four constant domains on the H and L chains (in contrast with the three found on IgG, IgA, and IgD); therefore, its pentamer form has the highest molecular weight of the immunoglobulins.

B. Functional properties (see Table 4.2). IgM, the earliest antibody to appear after antigenic stimulus, fixes complement avidly.

IV IgA

A. Structural properties (see Table 4.1)

1. **Forms.** IgA exists in three forms: a **monomer**, a **dimer** (in which a J chain joins two monomers; Figure 4.4), and a **dimer plus a secretory piece.**
   a. The dimer is transported across respiratory and intestinal mucosal barriers into the lumen by the secretory piece, which is a receptor for the IgA Fc region (**FcαR**) on the mucosal epithelium.
   b. The secretory piece also protects IgA from proteolysis.
2. The **structural designation** is $(\alpha_2\kappa_2)$ or $(\alpha_2\lambda_2)$ as the monomer, and $(\alpha_2\kappa_2)_2$ or $(\alpha_2\lambda_2)_2$ as the dimer.
3. **Two subclasses** exist: α_1 and α_2.

B. Functional properties (see Table 4-2)

1. **Serum half-life and concentration.** IgA is found in high concentrations in secretions; in serum, IgA exists mainly as a dimer with a half-life of 5 days.

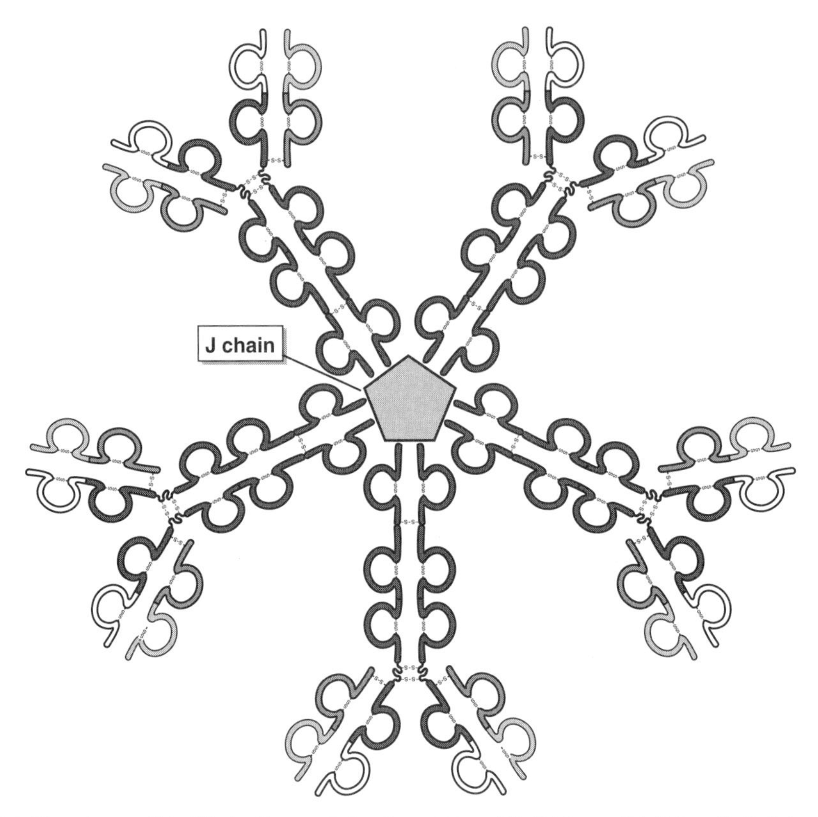

● **Figure 4.3** IgM pentamer. (Modified with permission from Abbas AK, Lichtman AH, Pober JS: *Cellular and Molecular Immunology,* 3rd ed. Philadelphia, WB Saunders, 1997, p 48.)

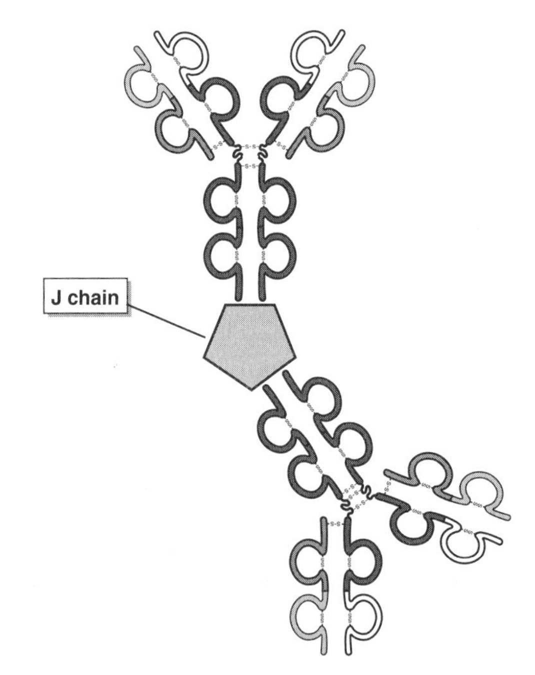

● **Figure 4.4** IgA dimer. (Modified with permission from Abbas AK, Lichtman AH, Pober JS: *Cellular and Molecular Immunology,* 3rd ed. Philadelphia, WB Saunders, 1997, p 48.)

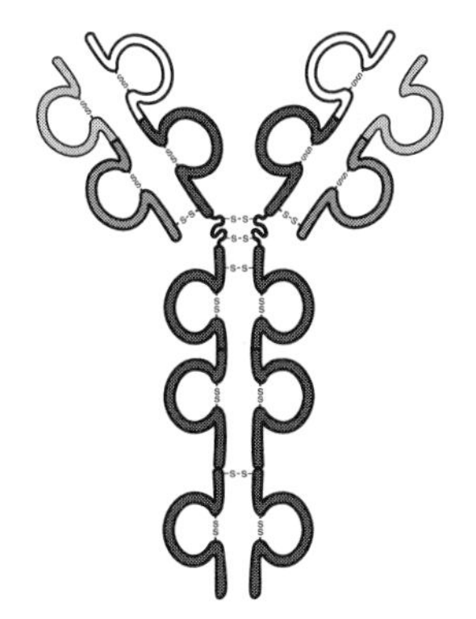

● **Figure 4.5** IgE. Note the four C domains. (Modified with permission from Abbas AK, Lichtman AH, Pober JS: *Cellular and Molecular Immunology,* 3rd ed. Philadelphia, WB Saunders, 1997, p 48.)

2. **Functions.** IgA is located in and protects mucosal tissues, saliva, tears, and colostrum by blocking bacteria, viruses, and toxins from binding to host cells.

V IgE

A. **Structural properties** (see Table 4.1)
   1. **Molecular weight.** IgE has four C domains (Figure 4.5) and a carbohydrate content of 18%, resulting in a molecular weight of 188,000 d.
   2. The **structural designation** for IgE is $\epsilon_2\kappa_2$ or $\epsilon_2\lambda_2$.
   3. The IgE molecule is unstable at 56°C and is called **reagin.**
   4. I14 mediates the B cell switch to IgE production.

B. **Functional properties** (see Table 4.2)
   1. **Serum concentration and half-life.** IgE has an extremely low serum concentration because its Fc region binds avidly to mast cells and basophils.
   2. **Functions**
      a. IgE adheres to tissue-bound mast cells and circulating basophils via Fcε receptors on these cells. The binding of antigen to these IgE-sensitized cells triggers the release of vasoactive amines (mainly histamine), resulting in **atopic disease** characterized by hives (a local reaction) and anaphylaxis (a systemic reaction).
      b. IgE does not cross the placenta or fix complement by the conventional pathway.
      c. The binding of IgE to Il-S–activated eosinophils results in elimination of parasitic helminths.
      d. Both total and allergen specific IgE can be quantified (see Chapter 6).

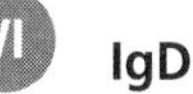

IgD

A. **Structural properties** (see Table 4.1). The structural formula for IgD is $\delta_2\kappa_2$ or $\delta_2\lambda_2$.

B. **Functional properties** (see Table 4.2)
   1. **Serum half-life and concentration.** IgD is found on the B cell membranes of 15% of newborns and again on adult peripheral blood lymphocytes in conjunction with IgM; serum levels are very low. The serum half-life is 2 to 3 days.
   2. **Functions.** IgD is a receptor on B cell membranes for antigen.

Chapter 5

Immunogenetics

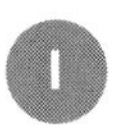

I GENETIC CONTROL OF IMMUNOGLOBULIN CHAIN SYNTHESIS

A. Genetic diversity. Human antibodies exhibit an enormous range ($\sim 10^8$) of specificities. The genetic basis for this diversity involves several factors:

1. **Different genes** code for the **variable** and **constant regions** of the heavy (H) and light (L) chains.
2. **Rearrangement of variable region and constant region genes during differentiation within the genome.** Any one of many different variable region genes can be linked to a single constant region gene, thus conserving DNA.
3. **Joining segment.** An additional gene sequence is required during the formation of the **L chain**. This sequence, the joining segment (J), joins the VL region gene to the CL region gene (Figure 5.1).
4. **Diversity segment.** An additional gene sequence is required during the formation of the **H chain**. This sequence, the **diversity segment**, links the VH gene to the J gene. These genes are then fused with the CH gene (Figure 5.2).
5. **H-chain class switching** from μ and δ to γ_3, γ_1, α_1, γ_2, γ_4, ϵ, and α_2 is dictated by a later rearrangement of the **class genes** in the CH region and is mediated by T cell cytokines (IL-4, IL-13, IFN-γ, TGF-β).

B. Random selection by each B cell from the variety of V, D, and J germ line genes available results in a large number of structural possibilities for the VL and VH epitope-binding regions of the immunoglobulins. This random selection is primarily responsible for the vast diversity of antibodies.

C. Allelic exclusion. Only one of the two parental alleles is expressed by a single B cell, resulting in a single H-chain isotype and L-chain subtype receptor capable of reacting with only one antigenic epitope.

II GENETIC CONTROL OF HUMAN LEUKOCYTE ANTIGENS (HLAs)

A. Functions of HLAs. HLAs control several elements, including:

1. **Discrimination** between self and nonself
2. **Antigen presentation** to T cells, but only of the same HLA type (self-MHC restriction)
3. **Susceptibility** to immunologic disorders and infectious agents (Table 5.1)

B. Classes of HLAs. HLAs are organized into three MHC classes of molecules (Table 5.2).

1. **Class I HLAs** are glycoproteins that are found on the **membranes of most nucleated cells.**
   a. **Gene regions.** Class I molecules are encoded by three gene regions: **A**, **B**, and **C**.
   b. **Function.** Class I molecules are linked to the cytotoxic T (Tc) cell through the CD8 molecule and present peptidic epitopes to **specific Tc receptors** (class I restriction). A single class I molecule can bind several different epitopes.

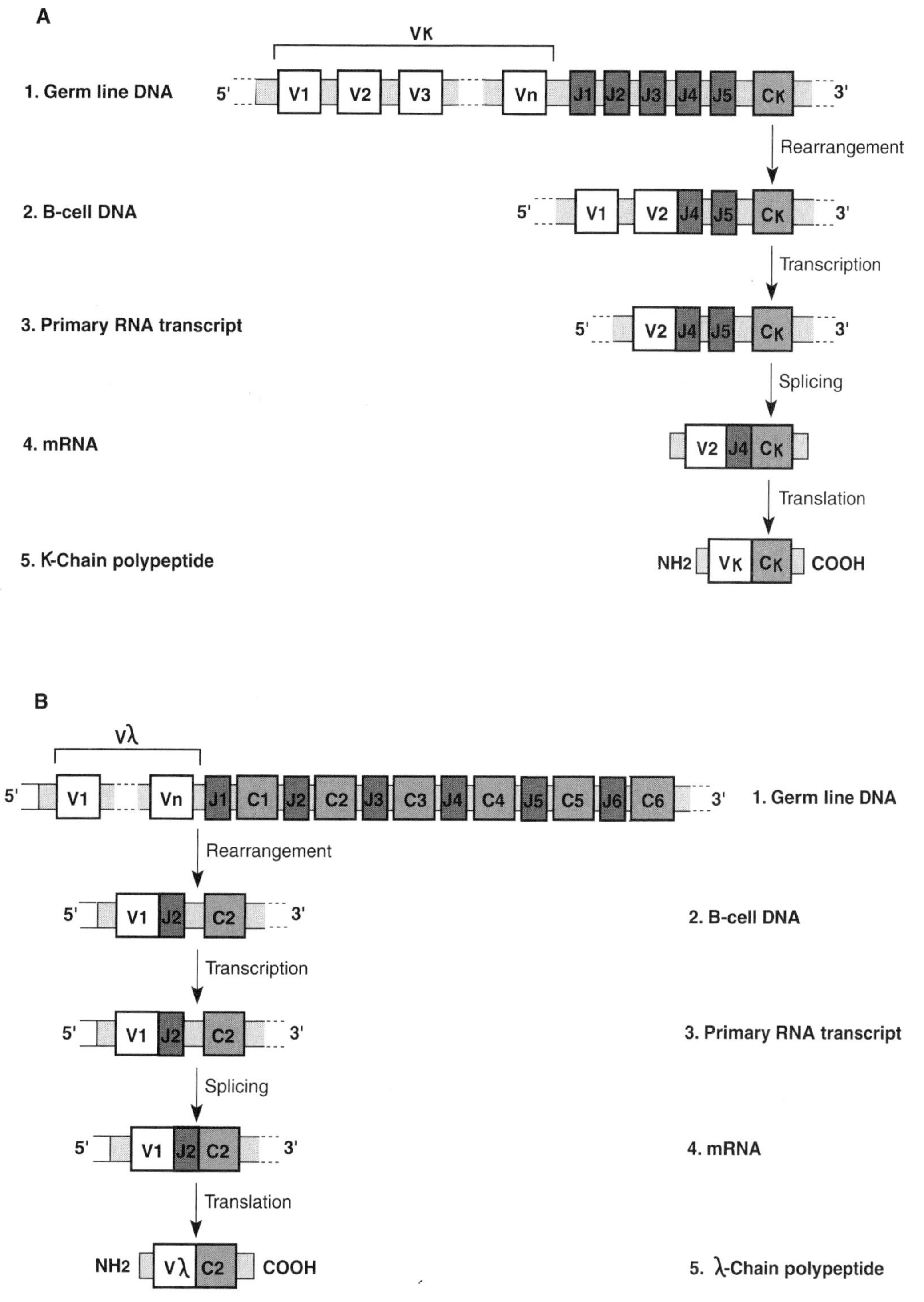

● **Figure 5.1** *(A)* Kappa (κ) light (L)-chain synthesis. From the pool of multiple variable *(V)* region genes on chromosome 2 in the germ line DNA *(1)*, one V region gene is joined to a joining *(J)* region gene, resulting in B-cell DNA *(2)*. Following removal of introns by recombinases, the primary RNA is transcribed *(3)*, resulting in mRNA *(4)* composed of one V region gene, one J gene, and the constant *(Cκ)* region gene. Translation of the mRNA results in the κ L-chain polypeptide *(5)*. (Redrawn with permission from Benjamini E: *Immunology: A Short Course*, 3rd ed. New York, Wiley-Liss, Inc., a subsidiary of John Wiley & Sons, Inc., 1996, p 98.) *(B)* Lambda (λ) L-chain synthesis. Rearrangement and synthesis of the λ L-chain genes occurs in an identical manner on chromosome 22, except for the availability of up to six Cλ exons for union to the VJ combined exon. This availability results in several subtypes.

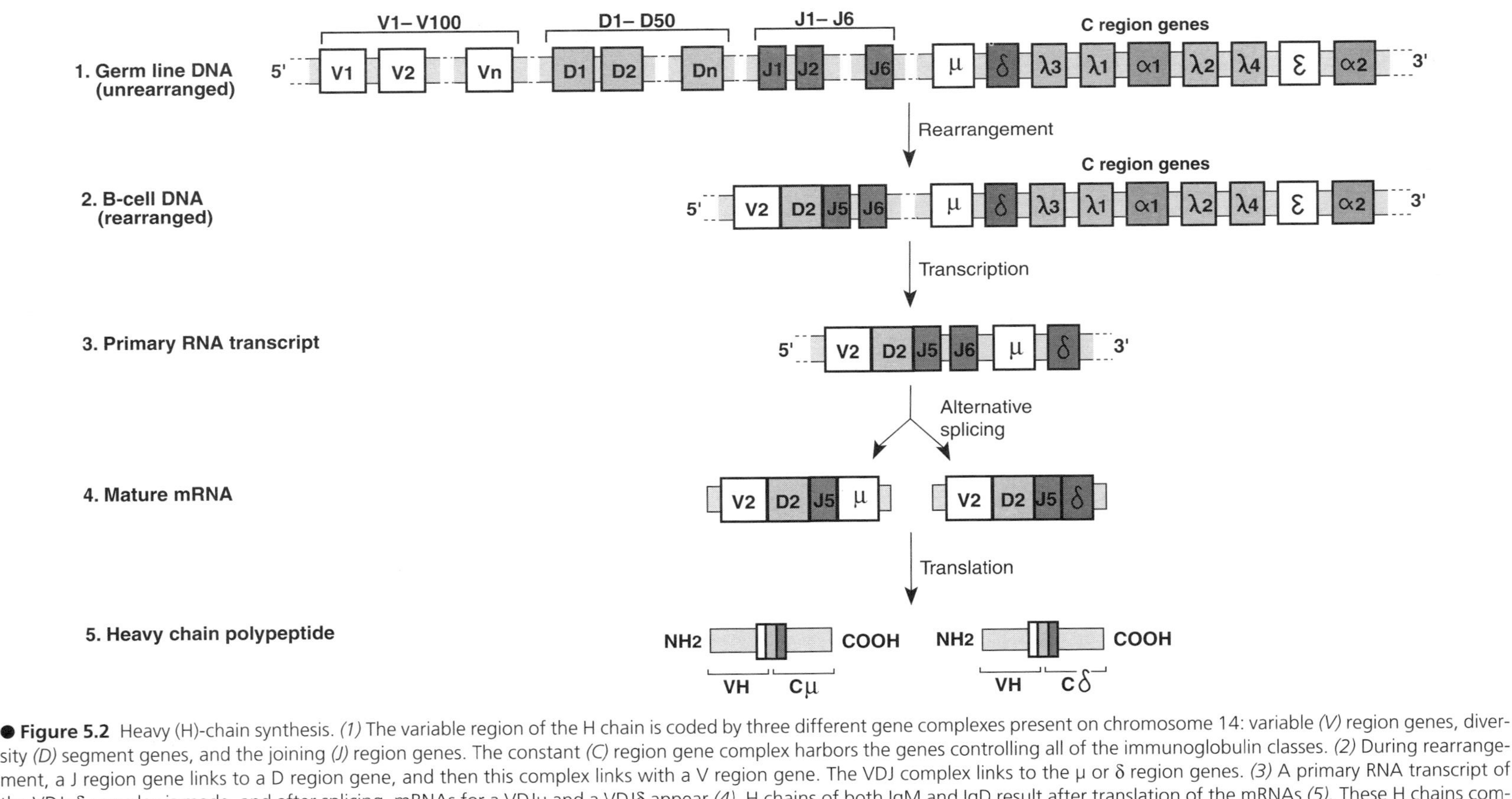

● **Figure 5.2** Heavy (H)-chain synthesis. *(1)* The variable region of the H chain is coded by three different gene complexes present on chromosome 14: variable *(V)* region genes, diversity *(D)* segment genes, and the joining *(J)* region genes. The constant *(C)* region gene complex harbors the genes controlling all of the immunoglobulin classes. *(2)* During rearrangement, a J region gene links to a D region gene, and then this complex links with a V region gene. The VDJ complex links to the μ or δ region genes. *(3)* A primary RNA transcript of the VDJμδ complex is made, and after splicing, mRNAs for a VDJμ and a VDJδ appear *(4)*. H chains of both IgM and IgD result after translation of the mRNAs *(5)*. These H chains combine with light (L) chains and deposit on the B cell membrane as the antigen receptors. Following antigen and cytokine stimulus, the IgM antibody is secreted (not illustrated). (Redrawn with permission from Benjamini E: *Immunology: A Short Course,* 3rd ed. New York, Wiley-Liss, Inc., a subsidiary of John Wiley & Sons, Inc., 1996, p 100.)

TABLE 5.1 ASSOCIATION OF HUMAN LEUKOCYTE ANTIGENS WITH DISEASE

Disorder	HLA Type	Risk*
Ankylosing spondylitis	B 27	87
Dermatitis herpetiformis	DR 3	56
Reiters syndrome	B 27	40
Insulin-dependent diabetes	DR 3/DR 4	33
Psoriasis vulgaris	C 6	13
Goodpasture's syndrome	DR 2	13
Rheumatoid arthritis	Dw 4/DR 4	10
Systemic lupus erythematosus	DR 3	5
Pernicious anemia	DR 5	5

*Times more likely to acquire the disorder than a person who does not have the specific HLA type.

c. **Structure** (Figure 5.3)
   (1) **Two chains** form the class I molecule.
      (a) The α **chain** has three external domains, a transmembrane segment, and a cytoplasmic tail.
      (b) The β_2-**microglobulin** is an invariant protein.
   (2) The **peptide-binding site**, found between domains α1 and α2, binds peptides containing 8–10 amino acids.

2. **Class II HLAs** are glycoproteins that are found on the **membranes of dendritic cells, macrophages,** and **activated T cells** and **B cells.**
   a. **Gene regions.** Class II molecules are encoded by three gene regions: **DP**, DQ, and **DR**.
   b. **Function.** Class II molecules are linked to the T helper (Th) cell through the CD4 molecule and present peptidic epitopes to **specific Th cell receptors** (class II restriction). A single class II molecule can bind several different epitopes.
   c. **Structure** (see Figure 5.3)
      (1) **Two chains,** α and β, form the class II HLA molecule. Each chain has two domains plus a transmembrane segment and cytoplasmic tail.
      (2) The **peptide-binding site,** formed by juxtaposition of the α1 and β1 domains, binds peptides containing 13–18 amino acids.

3. **Class III HLAs** control certain **serum proteins**, including several complement components and tumor necrosis factors (TNFs). Class III molecules are encoded by three gene regions: **C4**, **C2**, and **BF**.

TABLE 5.2 HUMAN LEUKOCYTE ANTIGEN (HLA) CLASSES

Complex	HLA							
MHC Class		I			II		III	
Region	B	C	A	DP	DQ	DR	C4, C2, BF	
Gene products	HLA-B	HLA-C	HLA-A	DP αβ	DQ αβ	DR αβ	C′ proteins	TNF-α TNF-β

From IMMUNOLOGY, 3/E by Janis Kuby. © 1992, 1994, and 1997 by W. H. Freeman and Company. Used with permission.
MHC = major histocompatibility complex; *TNF* = tumor necrosis factor.

A. Class I HLA molecule

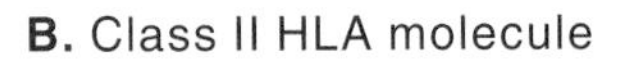

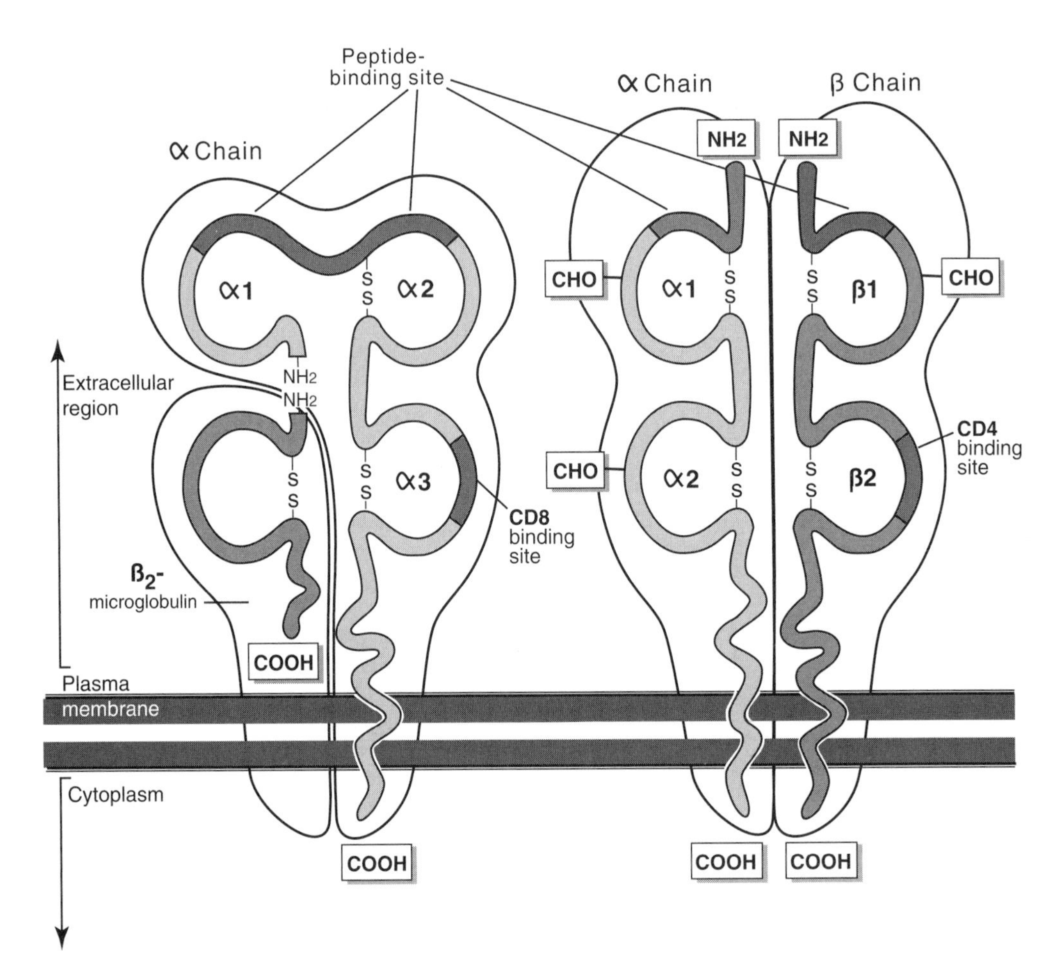

● **Figure 5.3** Structure of class I and class II human leukocyte antigen (HLA) molecules. *—SS—* = disulfide bond. (Redrawn with permission from Stites DP, Terr AI, Parslow TG: *Medical Immunology,* 9th ed. Stamford, CT, Appleton & Lange, 1997, p 86.)

C. Polymorphism

1. **Alleles.** Many alleles of class I and II molecules are present at each locus on chromosome 6 and are the major obstacles to organ transplantation.
2. **Haplotypes** from both parents are inherited and expressed codominantly.

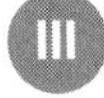

III GENETIC CONTROL OF THE T-CELL ANTIGENIC RECEPTOR (TCR)

A. Structure. The TCR is a **dimer** of either α and β chains (approximately 95%) or γ and δ chains (approximately 5%).

B. Function

1. In contrast to the monomeric IgM antigen receptor on the B-cell membrane, the **TCRs do not respond to soluble antigens.**
2. **TCRs recognize antigenic epitopes** only as peptidic fragments bound to either class I or class II HLA molecules on an antigen-presenting cell (APC) [e.g., dendritic cells, macrophages, B cells].

3. The **co-receptor, CD4 or CD8,** determines whether humoral immunity or cell-mediated immunity (CMI) occurs.
   a. Binding of the CD4 molecule to a class II HLA molecule on the APC results in **humoral immunity**.
   b. Binding of the CD8 molecule to a class I HLA molecule results in **CMI.**
4. Union of the specific TCR and co-receptor with the peptide–HLA membrane complex is associated with signal transduction into the cytoplasm by a complex of proteins. These proteins are collectively designated **CD3.**

C. **Genetic makeup**
1. Diversity among the TCRs is achieved through **gene rearrangements** similar to that of immunoglobulins (Figure 5.4).
2. Recombinase enzymes RAG-1 and RAG-2 are required for both heavy and light chain rearrangements in both early B and T cell antigen receptor expression.
3. RAG-1 and RAG-2 genes are part of an enzyme complex, the V (D) J recombinase in lymphocytes, which mediates the somatic recombination of V and J or V, D, J genes.
4. The phenomenon of **allelic exclusion** controls the genetic expression. Allelic exclusion occurs when only one of the parental alleles that code for the TCR is functional, rendering each T cell responsive to only a single epitope.

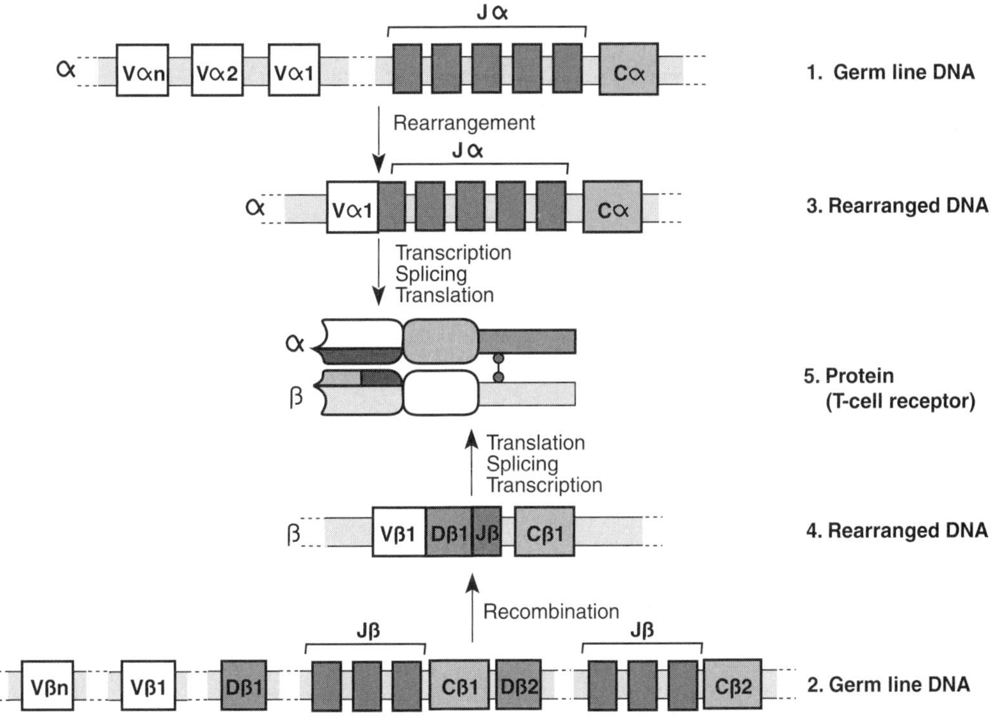

● **Figure 5.4** Synthesis of the human αβ T-cell receptor (TCR) genes. Synthesis of the γδ chains is thought to follow a similar pattern. *(1)* Multiple variable *(V)* region genes and joining *(J)* region genes occur at the TCRα locus on chromosome 14. *(2)* Similarly, multiple V region, diversity *(D)* segment, and J region genes occur at the TCRβ locus on chromosome 7. *(3)* During the rearrangement of α-chain genes, a randomly selected V gene is joined to a J gene and the exon is transcribed, combined with a constant *(Cα)* region gene, and translated. *(4)* Similarly, the β-chain exon is formed by the random linkage of a V region gene, first to a D region gene and a J region gene, and then to a Cβ gene. (Redrawn with permission from Janeway CA Jr, Travers P: *Immunobiology: The Immune System in Health and Disease.* New York, Garland Publishing, 1997, p 435.)

Chapter **6**

Immunologic Assays

OVERVIEW

A. Immunologic assays are sensitive and specific. Antigens, antibodies, antigen–antibody reactivity, cytokines, drugs, and cells can be detected in vitro or in vivo, some even in the nanogram and picogram range.

B. Ag–Ab reactions. The union of antigen with antibody is **specific** and **firm**, but **reversible**; multiple short-range forces are involved.

1. **Binding** occurs in seconds but is not visible until a **lattice** forms, which occurs more slowly. Since antibodies are bivalent, they form the lattice through cross-linkages (Figure 6.1). The composition of the lattice depends on the ratio of antigen to antibody.
   a. **Affinity** measures the binding energy between an antibody and a univalent epitope.
   b. **Avidity** is the total binding energy between an antibody and a multivalent antigen.
2. **Specificity** of Ag–Ab reactions is extreme. Changing the position of atoms, double bonds, structural conformation, or the composition of amino acids or sugars of the epitope changes specificity.

II PROTECTION TESTS

PROTECTION TESTS are used to determine the potency of vaccines.

A. Active. Following immunization with the vaccine that is being tested, groups of animals are challenged with increasing numbers of microorganisms. The lowest number of microorganisms lethal for 50% of the animals (i.e., the LD_{50}) is determined and compared to the LD_{50} in nonvaccinated animals to measure the protective power of the vaccine.

B. Passive. Graded amounts of serum from immunized individuals are transferred to normal animals, which are then challenged with the infectious agent. The highest dilution of serum effective at protecting 50% of the animals (i.e., ED_{50}) is determined as a measure of the efficacy of the vaccine.

III AGGLUTINATION TESTS

AGGLUTINATION TESTS are used to detect antibody union with large, particulate antigens.

A. Slide agglutination (qualitative)

1. **Blood grouping.** Slide agglutination is used in blood grouping to determine whether the donor's cells or serum possess antigens or antibodies reactive with the recipient's serum or cells.
   a. **Major crossmatch** uses the donor's cells plus the recipient's serum to determine whether anti–red blood cell (RBC) antibodies are present in the recipient's serum. Rapid clumping of the donor's cells will occur in vivo if anti-donor RBCs are present.
   b. **Minor crossmatch** uses the donor's serum plus the recipient's cells. Agglutination of the recipient's cells occurs if anti–RBC antibodies are

present in the donor's serum. However, a transfusion reaction under these conditions would be much less severe than one associated with a major crossmatch because the amount of antibodies transfused in the donor's serum is minimal relative to the number of RBCs in the recipient.

2. **Rapid identification of bacteria.** Bacteria can be identified by mixing a loopful of bacteria from the patient's culture with a battery of specific antibacterial antisera and noting which antiserum causes agglutination.

B. **Tube agglutination (semi-quantitative).** The killed microorganism suspected of causing the disease is added to dilutions of the patient's serum. The highest dilution that results in visible agglutination is called the **titer.** A **fourfold increase** in titer is necessary for diagnosis, owing to low levels of "natural" antibodies occurring in most normal human beings.

C. **Hemagglutination**

1. **Viral.** Myxoviruses (e.g., influenza, mumps, some pox viruses, and arboviruses) *spontaneously* agglutinate RBCs. This reaction is blocked in the presence of specific antiviral antibody. The patient's serum titer is determined by dilution.

2. **Coombs' test.** Weak or nonagglutinating anti–RBC antibody (generally Rh) can be detected by adding **antihuman immunoglobulin** to the RBC–anti-RBC complex.

   a. **Direct test.** Nonagglutinating Rh antibody attached in utero to the fetal or newborn Rh+ RBCs can be revealed by adding antihuman immunoglobulin directly to the infant's RBCs.

   b. **Indirect test.** Non-agglutinating anti-Rh antibodies in the maternal circulation can be detected by adding the mother's serum to Rh+ RBCs in vitro. The addition of antihuman immunoglobulin results in agglutination of the sensitized RBCs.

3. **Cold agglutination.** IgM complement–fixing antibodies, which agglutinate RBCs at temperatures below 37°C, are detected by incubation at lower temperatures. These antibodies are frequently autoimmune in nature and occur commonly in patients with primary atypical pneumonia caused by *Mycoplasma pneumoniae.*

IV

PRECIPITATION REACTIONS are used to detect soluble proteins and polysaccharides.

A. **Quantitative precipitin test.** This test measures either antigen or antibody in serum with analytical precision.

1. Increasing amounts of antigen are added in separate tubes containing a constant amount of the patient's serum.

2. The resulting precipitate in each tube is washed and analyzed by micromethods, and the precipitated antibody is plotted as a function of antigen added. **Three zones** result: **antibody excess, equivalence, and antigen excess** (Figure 6.1).

B. **Gel diffusion**

1. **Double diffusion (Ouchterlony test).** This technique detects impurities and identifies antigens in a mixture.

   a. Antigen and antibody diffuse toward each other from wells cut in 1% agar, forming a line of precipitate on contact.

   b. The number of lines reflects the number of antigens with different diffusion coefficients in a mixture (Figure 6.2).

2. **Immunoelectrophoresis** is used to identify immunologic disorders. Components of an antigen mixture are separated in agar first by migration in an electric field, followed by diffusion and subsequent precipitation with specific antibody diffusing from an overhead trough (Figure 6.3).

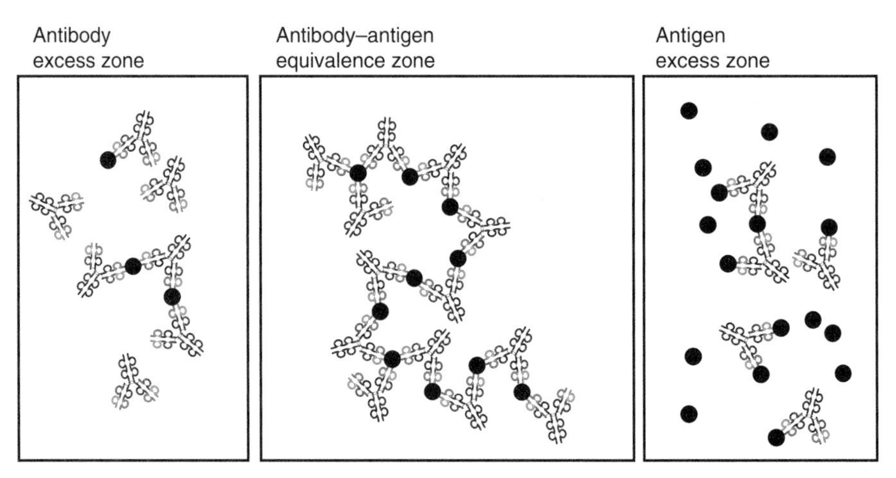

● **Figure 6.1** The size of antigen–antibody (Ag–Ab) complexes is determined by the ratio of antigen to antibody. In vivo, larger complexes (in antibody excess and at equivalence) are phagocytosed; smaller complexes (in antigen excess) escape and lodge in blood vessels and behind the renal basement membrane, causing vasculitis and glomerulonephritis.

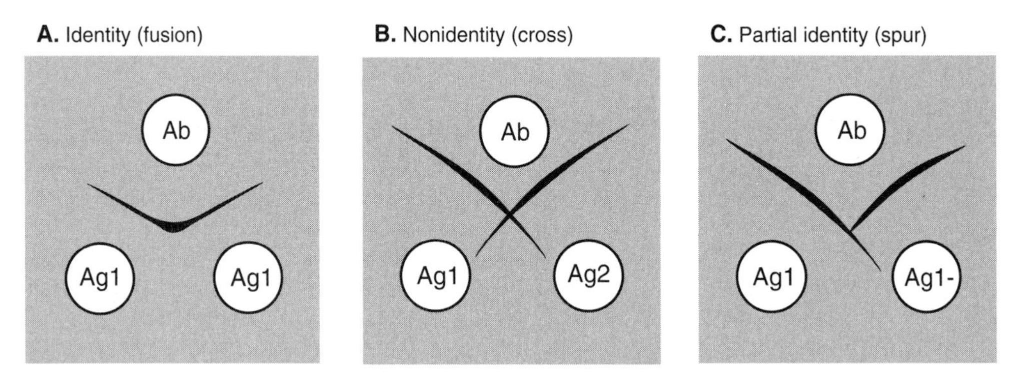

● **Figure 6.2** Agar-gel diffusion (Ouchterlony technique). To identify an unknown antigen, a sample containing the unknown is placed in a well adjacent to a well containing the suspected known antigen. A third well contains antibodies against each. As the antigens and antibodies diffuse through the gel, they form lines of precipitate on contact. Should the lines fuse as in *(A),* the unknown antigen is identified with the known; if the lines cross as in *(B),* the two are not identical; and if partial fusion occurs as in *(C),* one antigen has an additional epitope. The presence of additional lines of precipitation in the agar indicates a mixture of antigens in the unknown. *Ab* = antibody; *Ag* = antigen. (Redrawn with permission from Sell S: *Immunology, Immunopathology and Immunity,* 5th ed. Stamford, CT, Appleton & Lange, 1996, p 111.)

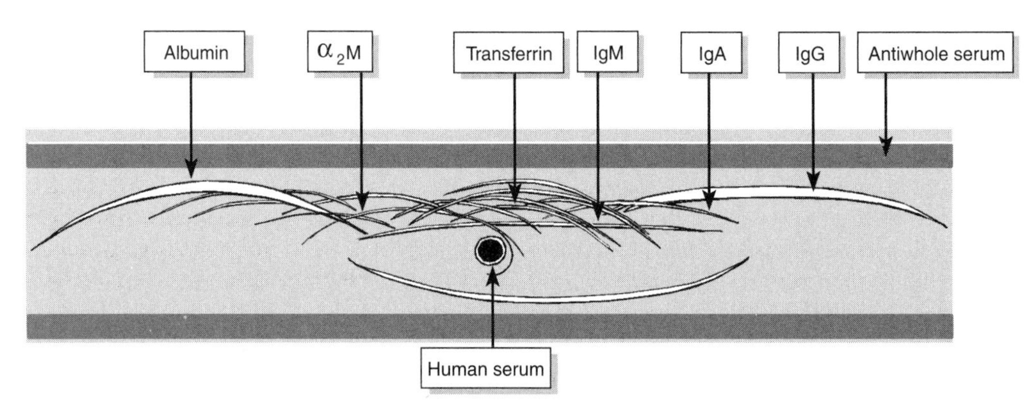

● **Figure 6.3** Immunoelectrophoresis. The antigenic components of human serum in the center well are separated according to their electrical charge in an electric field. Diffusion in agar is followed by precipitation with their respective antibodies diffusing from a central trough. The component immunoglobulins are identified. IgE and IgD concentrations are too low to be detected by this technique.

C. **Radioimmunoassay (RIA)** is based on the displacement of a known, radiolabeled antigen from an Ag–Ab complex by an unknown, unlabeled antigen (e.g., hormone) in a patient's body fluids. The extent of loss of the labeled antigen from the Ag–Ab complex can be measured and is a function of the concentration of the unknown antigen in the patient's fluid. Sensitivity is less than 1 ng.

D. Radioimmunosorbent test (RIST)
   1. Used to measure *total* IgE (non-specific) in an allergic patient's serum.
   2. The patient's serum is added to rabbit anti-human IgE, which has been adsorbed onto particulate (agarose) beads, and the complex is washed.
   3. I^{125} labelled rabbit anti human IgE is added, again washed, and the amount of radioactivity quantified, which reflects the total concentration of IgE in the patient's serum.

E. Radioallergosorbent test (RAST)
   1. Used to measure IgE in patient's serum *specific* for a given allergen.
   2. The suspected allergen is coupled to an insoluble matrix, the patient's serum added, and washed.
   3. I^{125} labelled rabbit anti-human IgE is added, the complex washed, and the bound radioactivity quantified, reflecting the serum level of IgE specific for that allergen.

F. **Enzyme-linked immunosorbent assay (ELISA)**
   1. **Antibody detection** is useful in detecting antibodies in low concentrations in a patient's serum (e.g., HIV).
      a. Dilutions of the test antibody solution are added to antigen adsorbed onto plastic wells. The complex is washed, and an enzyme-conjugated, anti-isotype antibody is added.
      b. After washing, the enzyme substrate is added.
      c. The resulting color is measured using a spectrophotometer. The titer is recorded as the highest dilution of antibody giving a color above the background.
   2. **Antigen detection** is useful for measuring nanogram (ng) amounts of hormones, drugs, and serum proteins.
      a. Dilutions of antigen are added to antibody that is adsorbed onto plastic wells. The resulting complex is washed, and an enzyme-conjugated antibody specific for a different epitope on the test antigen is added.
      b. After washing, the enzyme substrate is added, and the colored reaction is measured using a spectrophotometer. The titer is recorded as the highest dilution of antigen giving a color above the background.
   3. The use of an enzyme label eliminates problems associated with radioisotope disposal.

V COMPLEMENT FIXATION

A. **Complement system.** Complement (C′) fixation results in **cell lysis** and release of chemotactic factors C′3a and C′5a and requires **nine major factors** (**C′1–C′9**); most have enzymatic functions. Complement is fixed via **two pathways** (Figure 6.4).
   1. **Classical pathway.** Binding of the proenzyme C′1 to an Ag–Ab complex triggers a sequential reaction that results in cell lysis.
      a. IgM or a doublet of IgG bound to a cell surface antigen activates C′1qrs, which cleaves C′4 and C′2.
      b. Fragments C′4a and C′2a bind to the cell surface as C′4b2a, becoming a C′3 convertase that cleaves C′3 into two fragments, C′3a and C′3b.
      c. C′3b complexes with C′4b2a to become a C′5 convertase, which cleaves C′5 to C′5a and C′5b.

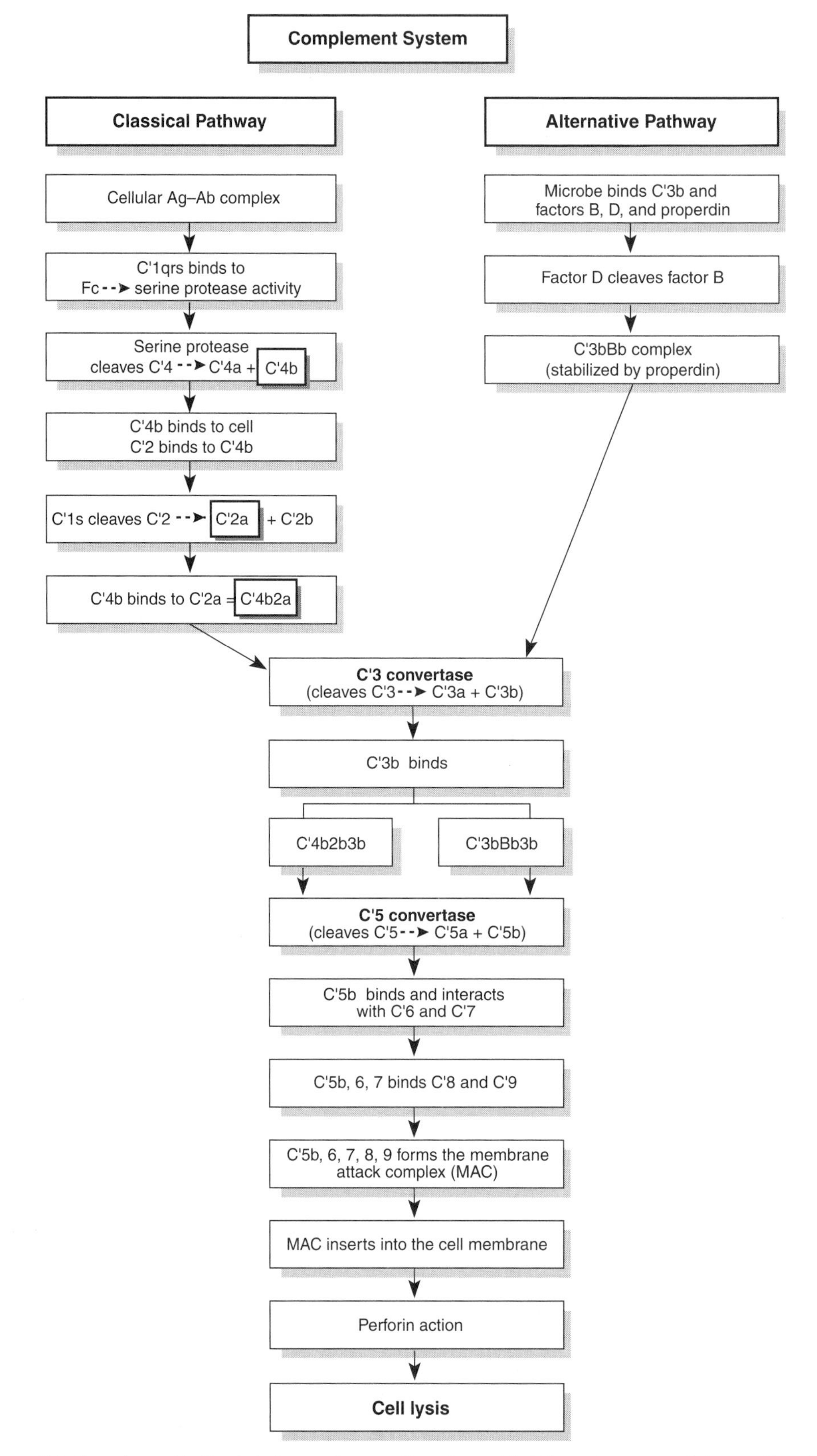

● **Figure 6.4** Complement is fixed via two pathways. Complement is lytic and promotes inflammation via its side products, C′3a and C′5a. A receptor for C′3 fragments on phagocytic cells promotes the phagocytosis of Ag–Ab–C′ complexes. *Ab* = antibody; *Ag* = antigen; *C′* = complement.

d. C′5b combines with C′6 and C′7 and inserts into the cell membrane.

e. C′8 and C′9 combine with the C′5b, 6, 7 complex to form the **membrane attack complex (MAC)**, resulting in cell lysis.

2. **Alternative pathway.** This pathway is activated by cell walls of certain bacteria, yeasts, and aggregated IgA. It does not require antibody or C′1, C′4, or C′2.

a. The cell walls bind to C′3b, which exists in normal serum. This complex binds with three other serum factors (B, D, and properdin), leading to a C′3 convertase. C′3bBb generates additional C′3b.

b. A C′3bBbC′3b complex forms, which becomes a C′5 convertase leading to the reactions that result in the MAC.

B. **Complement fixation test.** When specific antibody combines with its antigen, complement is bound and its serum concentration diminished. The extent of diminution can be measured in a complement fixation test and reflects the extent of antigen–antibody union.

VI FLUORESCENT ANTIBODY.

FLUORESCENT ANTIBODY. An antibody of concern is conjugated with **fluorescein isothiocyanate** or another dye that fluoresces under ultraviolet light. This can be used as a reagent to permit the visualization of either antigens or antibody in cells or tissues.

A. **Direct technique.** Fluorescinated antibody is added directly to the specimen (e.g., tissue) containing antigen and visualized under ultraviolet light.

B. **Sandwich technique**

1. If detection of the antigen in a specimen is desired, antibody is added, followed by fluorescinated anti-immunoglobulin antibody, and the specimen is visualized under ultraviolet light.
2. If detection of antibody in a specimen is desired, antigen is added, followed by fluorescinated antibody against the antigen, and the specimen is visualized under ultraviolet light.

VII WESTERN BLOT

A. This technique is widely used as a **confirmatory test for AIDS.** The patient's serum is added to known HIV antigens bound to a nitrocellulose matrix. A positive reaction is detected by the addition of a labeled, antihuman immunoglobulin antibody, as in the indirect ELISA test.

B. To **identify an antigen** in a mixture, the components of the mixture are separated by electrophoresis on a sodium dodecyl sulfate-polyacrylamide gel and "blotted" onto a nitrocellulose matrix. Labeled, known antibody is added to locate and identify the antigen of interest.

VIII CELL COUNTING AND FLOW CYTOMETRY

A. Microscopic analysis allows for visual inspection of cells to detect unusual morphologies and confirm information from automated methods.

1. Vital dyes such as trypan blue highlight cells and nuclei; heavily stained nuclei indicate cell death
2. Eosin methylene blue dye is used to detect and enumerate PMN subtypes (eosinophils, basophils, and neutrophils).

B. Flow cytometry counts every cell in a sample by sending a stream of single cells in a line through the beam on a laser. Any distortion of the light beam is detected by a high-powered detector, photomultiplier tube, and is recorded as an event. The flow cytometer can discriminate different objects or cells depending on size or granularity (i.e., secretory vesicles and multinuclei), cell viability, and cell type.

TABLE 6.1 SELECT CD ANTIGENS ON IMMUNE CELLS

CD antigen	Cells	Functions
CD1	DC	MHC class I like, presents lipid antigen
CD2	T cells NK cells Thymocytes	Adhesion molecule that binds CD58 controls Lck in T cell activation
CD3	T cells Thymocytes	Signal transduction associated with TCR
CD4	T_h1 and T_h2 cells Monocytes Macrophages	Co-receptor that docks to MHC class II and controls Lck in T cell activation
CD8	Cytotoxic T cells	Co-receptor that docks to MHC class I and controls Lck in T cell activation
CD11 (a–d)	a) Lymphocytes Granulocytes Monocytes Macrophage	αL subunit to integrin LFA-1 binds to CD54, CD50, and CD102
	b) Myeloid cells NK cells	αM subunit of integrin CR3 and binds fibrinogen
	c) Myeloid cells	αX subunit of integrin CR4 and binds fibrinogen
	d) Leukocytes	αD subunit of integrin
CD14	DC Macrophage	TLR, binds LPS binding protein
CD16	Neutrophils NK cells Macrophages	Subunit of low-affinity Fc receptor and mediates endocytosis
CD18	Leukocytes	Integrin β2 subunit, associates with CD11(a–d)
CD19	B cells	Subunit of co-receptor for BCR complex and binds protein tyrosine and PI-3 kinases
CD21	B cells	Subunit of co-receptor for BCR complex
CD23	Eosinophils B cells Macrophage	Low-affinity receptor for IgE
CD25	Activated T cells and B cells Macrophage	α subunit of IL-2 receptor
CD28	T cells Activated B cells	T cell activation and receptor for co-stimulatory signal by binding CD80 and CD86
CD34	Hematopoietic stem and Progenitor cells Endothelium	Receptor for CD62L, a selectin
CD35	B cells Monocytes Neutrophils Eosinophils DC	Complement receptor 1 and mediates phagocytosis

TABLE 6.1 SELECT CD ANTIGENS ON IMMUNE CELLS (*continued*)

CD antigen	Cells	Functions
CD45	All hematopoietic cells	Transmembrane tyrosine phosphatase, regulates Src kinases and augments lymphocyte activation
CD54	Ubiquitous to all cells	Intracellular adhesion molecule (ICAM) binding CD11a and CD11b
CD56	NK cells	Adhesion molecule
CD58	Ubiquitous to all cells	Adhesion molecule, binds CD2
CD82L	B cells T cells Monocytes NK cells	Leukocyte adhesion molecule, mediates rolling interaction with endothelium
CD64	Monocytes Macrophages	High affinity receptor for IgG
CD71	Ubiquitous to all Proliferating cells (i.e., activated cells)	Transferrin receptor
CD80	B cells	Co-stimulator and ligand for CD28 and CTLA-4
CD81	Lymphocytes	Subunit of B cell co-receptor
CD86	Monocytes Activated B cells DC	Co-stimulator and ligand for CD28 and CTLA-4
CD89	Leukocytes	IgA receptor

1. Vital dyes such as propidium iodine will label chromatin in dead or dying cells. Cells fixed with ethanol (80%) will completely take up dye to provide a differential count of cell morphologies or cell cycle. Dye added to a sample of living cells will discriminate between living and dead cells.
   a. Cell morphology can be used to detect cells having more cytoplasm (macrophage and neutrophils) versus those with lesser cytoplasm (lymphocytes).
   b. Cell cycle analysis is a function of the dye loading per cell. Cells proceeding through mitosis will accumulate more dye as the amount of chromatin increases. All circulating lymphocytes should be at interphase; cells showing mitosis are indicative of leukemia.
2. Antibodies conjugated with fluorescent dyes can be used to tag cells expressing a specific protein. The most common proteins tagged for flow cytometry are membrane CDs (see Table 6.1).
   a. Single tagging can identify a class of cells; for example, B cells express surface immunoglobulin, T cells express CD3.
   b. Multiple tagging provides for a more refined search to discriminate subtypes; for example, helper T cells express both CD3 and CD4, cytotoxic T cells express CD3 and CD8.

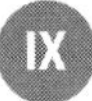

IX REVERSE TRANSCRIPTION POLYMERASE CHAIN REACTION (RT-PCR)

RT-PCR is a highly sensitive procedure that identifies the presence of protein based on the assumption that mRNA levels are an indication of protein expression. This method will identify minute quantities of substances from blood samples such as cytokines, receptors, and virus. The production of cytokines from only a few cells in a whole blood sample can be readily detected.

X DNA MICROARRAYS

This is a method to screen immune cells for the differential expression of a large number of different genes. This method allows for the identification of mutated genes in immune cells (e.g., p53, ras, c-myc, and Bcl-2) and can be used to diagnosis diseases.

Chapter 7

The Immune Response

I

HUMORAL IMMUNITY is mediated by antibodies that protect the body fluids (Figure 7.1).

A. Antigen entry

1. If antigen entry is **intravenous**, the antigen is phagocytized or pinocytosed in the **spleen**.
2. If antigen entry is **other than intravenous**, the antigen moves to the **lymph node**, draining the site of entry.

B. Antigen processing. In the lymph nodes or spleen, the antigen encounters the **T cell, B cell, antigen-presenting cell (APC) triad** and is initially processed by the APC (Figure 7.2). Antigen processing results in the activation of T cells.

1. **Viruses and intracellular parasite antigens**
   a. These antigens are **synthesized endogenously** within the APC cytoplasm and endoplasmic reticulum, then processed to peptides by proteasomes.
   b. The **resulting peptides** bind to the heavy chains of **major histocompatibility complex (MHC) class I** molecules and migrate to the APC membrane, where they are presented to CD8+ T cells (Figure 7.3A).
2. **Exogenous protein antigens**
   a. These antigens enter the APC from the **extracellular environment** by pinocytosis and are processed in acidic endosomal vacuoles.
   b. The **resulting peptides** bind to the cleft in **MHC class II** molecules and are transported to the cell membrane, where they are presented to **CD4+** T cells (Figure 7.3B).

C. Activation of T and B cells

1. **Exogenous protein antigens.** After being transported to the APC cell membrane, the antigenic peptide–MHC class II complex is presented to CD4+ T helper (Th) cells (Figure 7.4A).
   a. **Th1 cell response.** Following activation, the CD4+ Th1 cell clone differentiates, divides logarithmically, and secretes **IL-2, IFN-γ,** and **TNF-α.**
      (1) IL-2 is necessary for T and B cell transformation.
      (2) IFN-γ
         (a) A **potent macrophage** and **natural killer (NK) cell activator,** IFN-γ enhances cell-mediated immunity (CMI).
         (b) IFN-γ **triggers HLA antigen presentation** by endothelial cells.
         (c) IFN-γ **downregulates IL-4 synthesis** by Th2 cells; thus, it can also suppress antibody formation.
      (3) TNF-α
         (a) Activates macrophages
         (b) Stimulates the acute-phase response
         (c) Synergizes with IL-1 in inducing the acute-phase response
   b. **Th2 cell response.** Following antigen activation and stimulation by IL-2, the CD4+ Th2 cell responds by transforming, differentiating, and dividing logarithmically, while secreting **IL-4, IL-5, IL-10,** and **IL-13.**

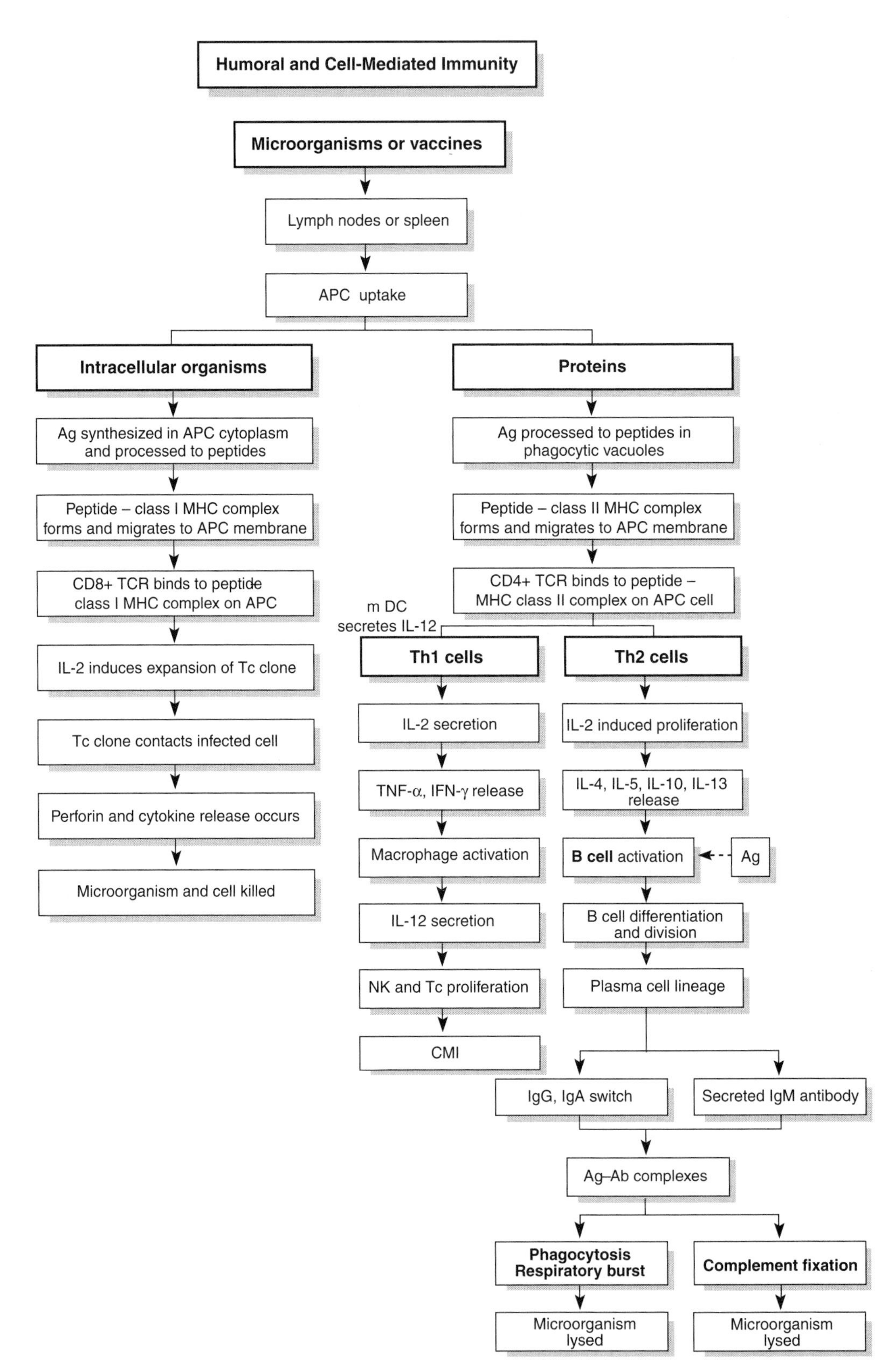

● **Figure 7.1** Humoral and cell-mediated immunity. *Ag–Ab* = antigen–antibody; *APC* = antigen-presenting cell; *CD* = cluster of differentiation; *IFN-γ* = interferon-γ; *Ig* = immunoglobulin; *IL* = interleukin; *MHC* = major histocompatibility complex; *Tc* = cytotoxic T cell; *TCR* = T-cell receptor; *TNF-α* = tumor necrosis factor-α.

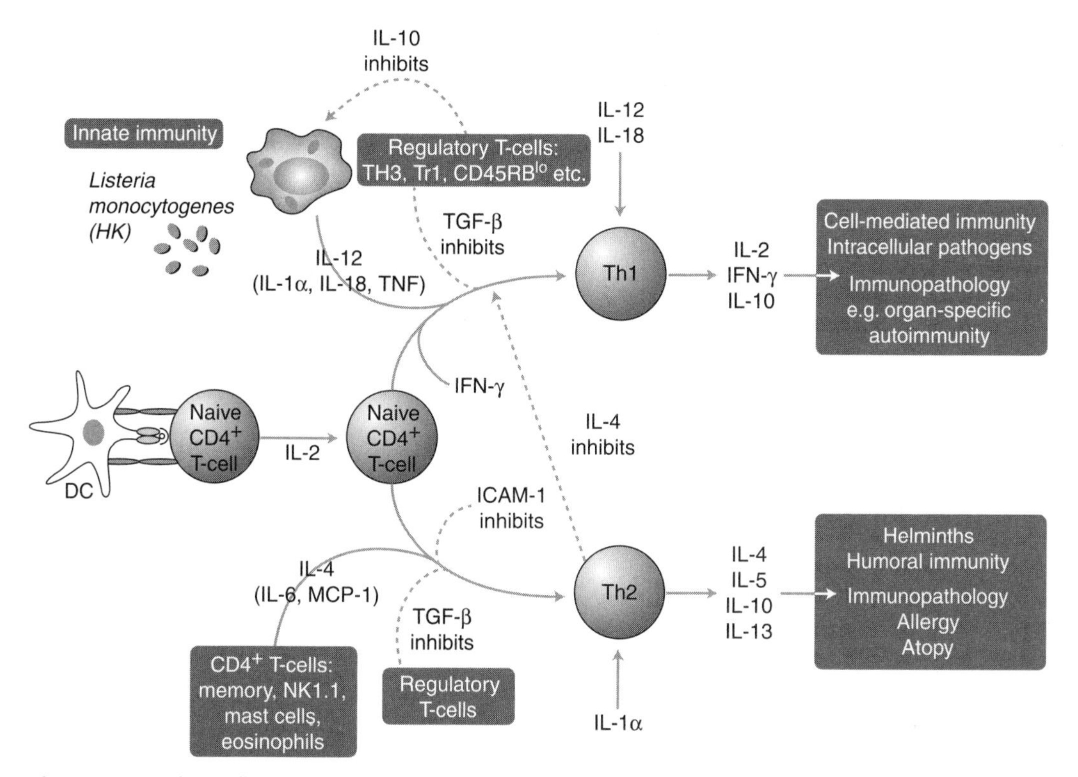

● **Figure 7.2** Dendritic cell regulation of T helper responses. (Modified with permission from O'Garra A, Arai N. The molecular basis of T helper 1 and T helper 2 cell differentiation. Trends Cell Biol 2000;10:546.) mDC activate naïve T cells (see Figure 3.1); however, subsequent T cell development into Th1 or Th2 may be regulated by other innate immune cells.

(1) **IL-4**
  (a) Favors the development of antibody synthesis by stimulating B-cell differentiation
  (b) Downregulates IFN-γ by Th1 cells and, thus, can suppress CMI
  (c) Is necessary for the switch to immunoglobulin E (IgE) production

(2) **IL-5**
  (a) Functions synergistically with IL-4 and IL-2 to help B-cell differentiation
  (b) Facilitates IgA synthesis
  (c) Stimulates the growth and differentiation of eosinophils

(3) **IL-10**, like IL-4, inhibits Th1 cell release of IFN-γ and IL-2, thereby negating macrophage activation by IFN-γ.

(4) **IL-13** mimics IL-4 actions, inhibiting Th1 cytokine release.

c. **B-cell response**

(1) Antigen selects the **clone of B cells** with the membrane-bound IgM antigen receptor that is specific for the antigen epitope.

(2) **Binding of antigen** along with **stimuli from the T cell cytokines IL-2 and IL-4** triggers differentiation of that B-cell clone into a **large blast cell**, and **logarithmic division** occurs.

(3) IL-5 continues this process, during which the B cell acquires the **cytoplasmic "machinery"** necessary for **antibody synthesis**.
  (a) **H and L chains** are synthesized, assembled, and, under IL-6 influence, terminal differentiation into a plasma cell and secretion of IgM occurs.

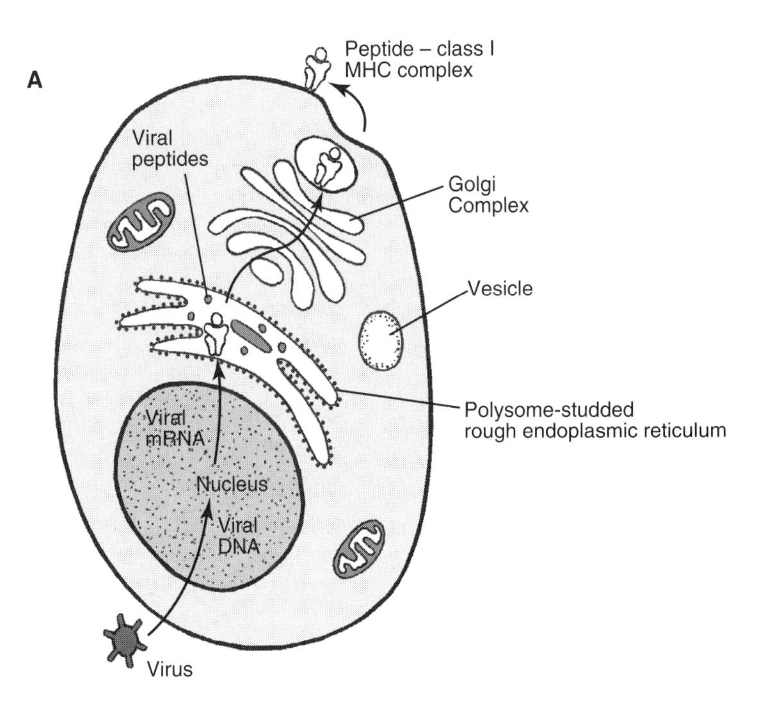

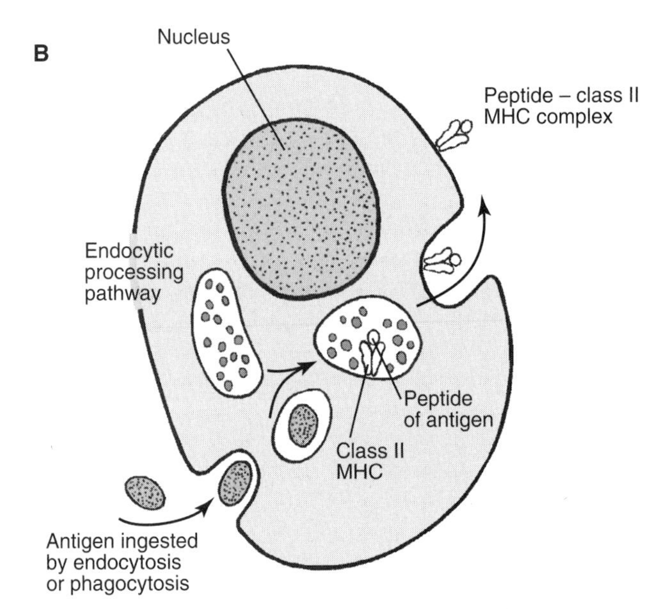

● **Figure 7.3** Antigen processing *(A)* of intracellular organisms and *(B)* of exogenous proteins. (From IMMUNOLOGY, 3/E by Janis Kuby. © 1992, 1994, and 1997 by W. H. Freeman and Company. Used with permission.)

(b) Subsequent **gene rearrangements** result in a switch to IgG, IgA, and IgE synthesis and secretion.
(i) IL-4 and IFN-γ influence the switch to IgG; TGF-β influences the switch to IgA; and IL-4 influences the switch to IgE.
(ii) The binding of CD40 on the B cell to its ligand on the Th cell (CD40L), is necessary for switching to occur.

d. **B memory cells.** Memory cells of all classes are generated independently of the **plasma cell** lineage. **These memory cells migrate to various lymphoid tissues**, where they have an extended survival.

e. **Secondary response.** Further exposure to the same antigen can result in the following:
(1) A shorter induction period to antibody synthesis
(2) More rapid class switching from IgM to IgG
(3) Increased IgG with antibodies of higher affinity
(4) Predominant IgA synthesis in mucosal tissues

2. **Viruses and intracellular parasite antigens.** Synthesized in the cytoplasm and transported to the APC membrane, the antigenic peptide–MHC class I complex is presented to CD8+ cytotoxic (Tc) cells (Figure 7.4B).

II **CELL-MEDIATED IMMUNITY (CMI)** is directed mainly against **intracellular-dwelling microorganisms** and **aberrant, endogenous cells** (e.g., cancers) (Figure 7.1).

A. **Mechanism.** Immune reactivity is effected by sensitized **T cells, macrophages**, and **NK cells** on direct contact with the target cell.

1. Reactivity is transferrable to **normal, nonsensitized hosts** with sensitized effector cells.
2. Antibody is not involved, except in **antibody-dependent cellular cytotoxic reactions (ADCC)**. In these cases, the effector cell is linked to the target cell by an antibody bridge, with the **Fab portion** binding to the specific membrane antigen on the target cell, and the **Fc portion** binding to the Fc receptor on an activated effector cell.

B. **Types of CMI**

1. **Reaction to infectious agents** (e.g., **tuberculin test**)

a. **Function.** The tuberculin test reveals immune reactions in internal organs (e.g., lungs).
(1) **Domestic use.** The tuberculin test is used in the United States to identify human beings exposed to, or actively infected with, *Mycobacterium tuberculosis*. The underlying principle can be extrapolated to apply to the detection of other intracellular microorganisms.
(2) **Foreign use.** Extensive use of bacille Calmette-Guérin (BCG) vaccine in other countries nullifies their use of the tuberculin test as a diagnostic test.

b. **Procedure.** A patient **previously exposed** to *M. tuberculosis* is injected intradermally with an extract of *M. tuberculosis* [called **purified protein derivative (PPD)**].

c. **Reaction process [delayed-type hypersensitivity (DTH)]**
(1) A contained lesion of **induration and erythema**, peaking in 1 to 2 days, results from the inflammatory response induced by sensitized T-cell action at the site of PPD deposition.
(2) The skin lesion is initiated by **Langerhans cell** presentation of antigen to previously sensitized delayed-type hypersensitivity T (TDTH) cells that have been recruited to the site of antigen deposition by chemokines.
(3) Subsequent APC– and T cell–secreted cytokines and chemokines attract **polymorphonuclear neutrophils (PMNs)**, followed by CD4+ T cells

and a dominant, nonspecific, perivascular accumulation of monocytic/macrophage cells.

(4) **Destruction of the organisms, tissue, or both** follows macrophage infiltration.

2. **Granulomatous reactions** occur if the antigen persists in the tissues and continues to stimulate host reactivity.
   a. **Chronic stimulation** by intracellular organisms releases chemotactic agents (e.g., IL-1, IL-8), leading to an inflammatory cell influx.
   b. **IL-4** and **IFN-γ** promote the retention of macrophages and cause the fusion of monocytes at the site, leading to an **epithelioid cell granuloma** derived from macrophages, histiocytes, and epithelioid cells.
3. **Contact dermatitis** occurs when small-molecular-weight chemicals (**haptens**) or irritants are deposited into the skin, causing a CMI reaction. **Common eliciting agents** include nickel, dinitrochlorobenzene, rubber, poison ivy, and poison sumac.
   a. The **haptenic agent** becomes antigenic by combining with intradermal proteins as carriers via NH_3 or S groupings. **Langerhans cells and endothelial cells** serve as APCs.
   b. **Subsequent reexposure** to the agent results in chemokine and cytokine release, monocytic/macrophage infiltration, and a **vesiculating lesion** with **erythema and induration.**

C. Consequences of CMI

1. Although CMI is basically a defense mechanism against foreign substances, **cells** in the vicinity of antigen deposition, as well as those harboring microorganisms, are damaged if the inflammatory response induced is excessive.
2. The **magnified inflammatory response** induced by activated macrophages, cytotoxic T (Tc) lymphocytes, and NK cells causes this damage.
   a. **Activated macrophages**
      (1) **Activation**
         (a) Macrophages are activated **nonspecifically**, primarily by **IFN-γ** released by Th1 cells following antigenic stimulation.
         (b) **Microbial products** [e.g., bacterial lipopolysaccharides (endotoxins)] also are potent macrophage activators; these substances induce TNF-α and IFN-γ release.
      (2) **Consequences.** Activation results in **increased phagocytosis** and **microbicidal action.**
         (a) **Microbial killing** occurs mainly through **reactive oxygen species** (H_2O_2, O_2^- anion, and nitric oxide).
         (b) Activated macrophages generate many other microbicidal factors [e.g., IL-1, tissue factor, thrombin, platelet-derived growth factor (PDGF), TGF-β, TNF-α, and prostaglandins].
   b. **Tc lymphocytes**
      (1) Macrophage secretion of IL-12 acts synergistically with IL-2 to induce the differentiation of Th1 and NK cells into **Tc cells.**
      (2) Tc cells are mainly of the CD8+ phenotype. Binding to a class I MHC molecule on the target cell is facilitated by **multiple coreceptors (see Figure 7.4B).**
      (3) Unlike the IgM B cell antigenic receptor, the TCR is not secreted; immunity must be effected by **contact** with the target cells (e.g., virus- and bacteria-infected cells; foreign transplants; antigenic tumors; autoimmune susceptible, endogenous cells).

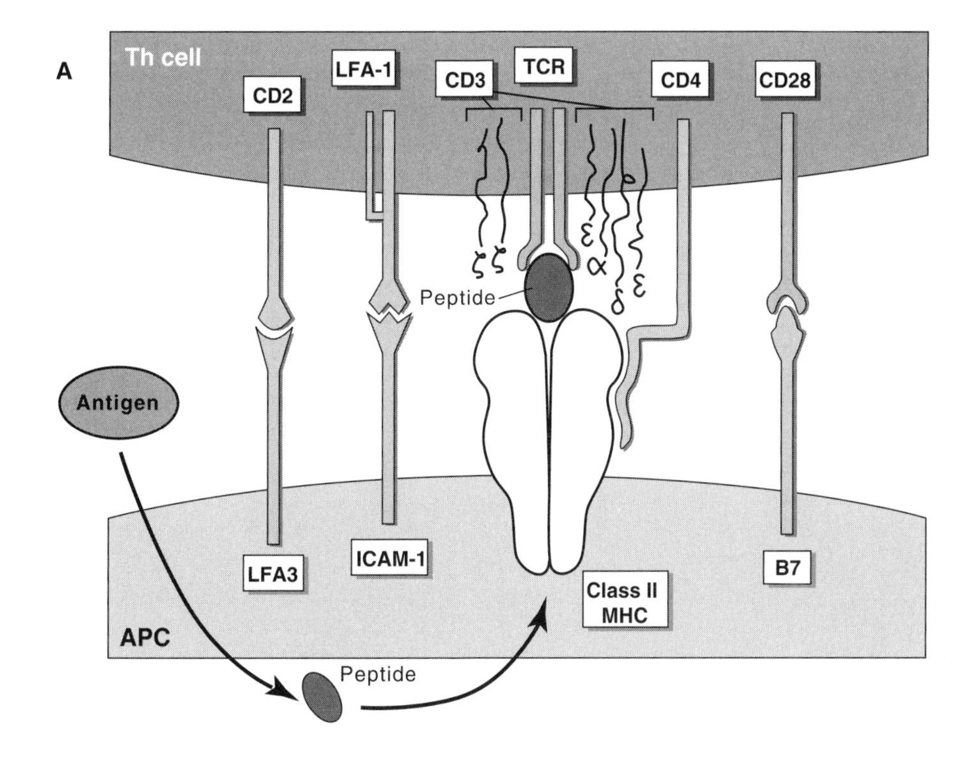

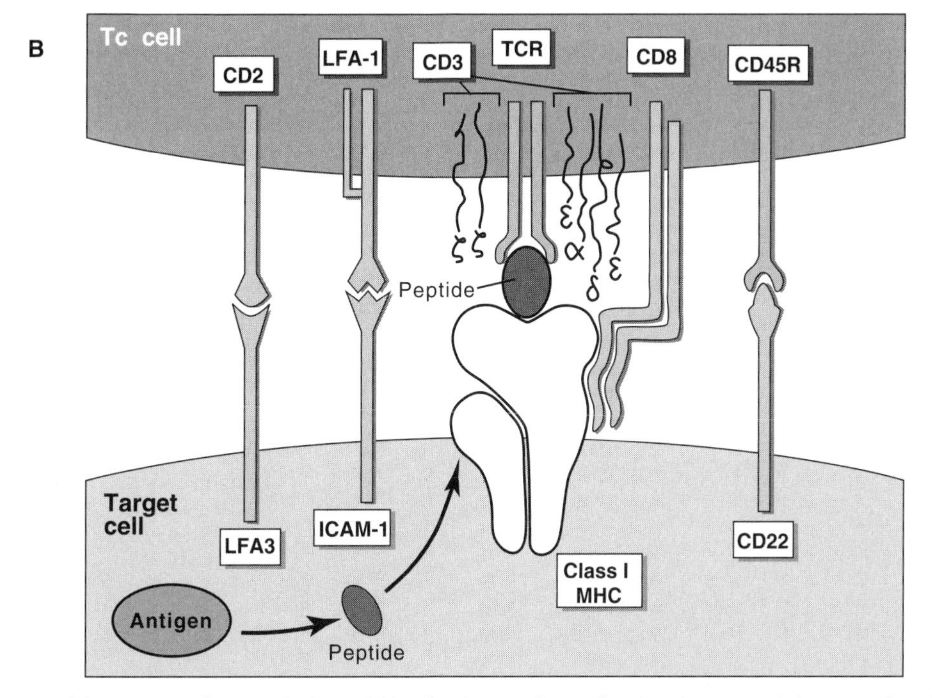

● **Figure 7.4** *(A)* Activation of a CD4+ helper T (Th) cells. The specific T-cell antigenic receptor ($\alpha\beta$:*TCR* or $\gamma\delta$:*TCR*) binds to the peptide–class II major histocompatibility complex *(MHC)* by the antigen-presenting cell *(APC)*. The CD4 molecule links to the MHC. An activation signal is transduced by the TCR–CD3 complex, which is composed of three polypeptides (α, δ, ε) and two ζ chains. Accessory T-cell adhesion molecules [e.g., CD2, leukocyte function–associated antigen-1 *(LFA-1)*, and CD28] facilitate adherence of the Th cell to the APC and influence interleukin-2 (IL-2) synthesis. *(B)* Activation of CD8+ cytotoxic T *(Tc)* cells. (From IMMUNOLOGY, 3/E by Janis Kuby. © 1992, 1994, and 1997 by W. H. Freeman and Company. Used with permission.)

(4) Following cell–cell contact, Tc lytic function emerges from **exocytosis of granzymes** (i.e., granules containing enzymes), **perforins**, **cytolysins**, **lymphotoxins**, and **serine esterases** (Figure 7.5).

c. **NK cells**

(1) **Function.** NK cells kill tumor cells and those infected by viruses, but they do not kill most normal cells. They are prominent in graft-versus-host reactions.

(2) **Morphology.** NK cells are large granular lymphocytes that contain antagonists similar to Tc cells.

(a) NK cells do not exhibit T-cell or B-cell phenotypes and lack CD3 and TCR markers.

(b) NK cells do not require prior sensitization to exhibit cytolysis, but they can be activated by IL-2, IL-12, and IFN-γ.

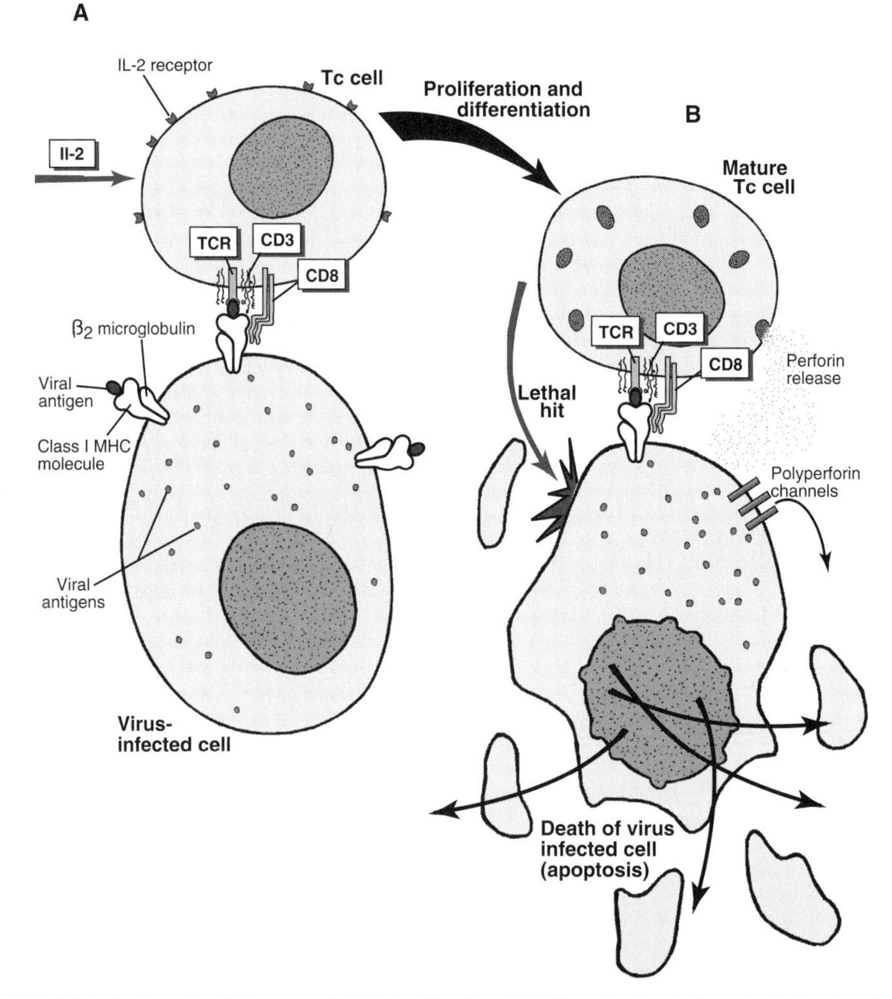

● **Figure 7.5** *(A)* Activation of a CD8+ cytotoxic T *(Tc)* cell leads to *(B)* killing of a virus-infected cell. The virus-infected cell synthesizes viral antigens, which, when processed, bind to major histocompatibility complex (*MHC*) class I. The viral peptide–MHC class I complex binds to the T cell antigenic receptor *(TCR),* triggering the Tc cells to proliferate and differentiate into mature Tc cells. *(B)* The mature Tc cells release perforin, which binds to the virus-infected cell via calcium ions. The perforin causes channels to form in the membrane of the virus-infected cell, causing the cell contents to leak out. The resultant osmotic imbalance causes the death of the virus-infected cell. (Modified with permission from Benjamini E: *Immunology: A Short Course,* 3rd ed. New York, Wiley-Liss, Inc., a subsidiary of John Wiley & Sons, Inc., 1996, p 212.)

Chapter **8**

Signal Transduction in Immune Cells

I EFFECTIVE IMMUNE RESPONSES REQUIRE COMMUNICATION BETWEEN A WIDE RANGE OF CELL TYPES

A. Regulating interactions between cells

1. Circulating lymphocytes are generally quiescent, but can be called up for duty once presented with antigen by APC. These lymphocytes, when activated, proceed through a programmed pattern of development. At any stage of development a lymphocyte can differentiate into a cell with newly acquired abilities or retire back into a quiescent state as a memory cell. Hence the immune system must be adaptable, while retaining an ability to develop exceptionally refined recognition systems. To maintain these traits, cells of the immune system must communicate effectively.

2. Innate immune cells regulate lymphocyte development by controlling three stages:

a. Recognize invading virus or bacteria as a foreign pathogen

b. Deliver the activation signals to a specific T cell

c. Translate that information and delivering the appropriate mix of cytokines to mount an adaptive immune response with lasting memory

3. Examples are:

a. APC stimulate T cells by an MHC restricted mechanism and deliver IL-12 to continue differentiation to T_h1 cells

b. The presence of IL-4 can cause activated T cells differentiation to T_h2 cells

B. Communication involves at least four systems: endocrine, paracrine, autocrine, and tactile messages that are transduced through membrane-bound receptors. In general, these receptors will have multimeric structures with recognition separate from signal transduction. Often the recognition structure is also multimeric, composed of a chain with high affinity properties and a second chain with low affinity properties. The low affinity chain is also generally shared with other receptor complexes leading to a redundancy in structure and function. The signal-transducing complexes also share homologies between different signaling activities. This sharing of "modules" permits the cell to have signaling components ready for use and needs to only express a new module to provide specificity (i.e., de novo expression of the IL-2α subunit dramatically shifts a cell's response to IL-2). In contrast, the presence of these low affinity complexes also plays an important role in pathology since dramatic rises in cytokines lead to nonspecific and often lethal states.

C. Signal transduction across a membrane requires a change in the receptor's conformation; either a shift in shape (i.e., heptahelical receptors) or an oligomerization of surface receptor modules. For the cytokine receptors there are several steps.

1. Cytokine binding causes receptors to cluster, typically a dimerization.

2. Receptor dimerization brings the cytosolic tails into close proximity.

3. Associated with the cytosolic tail is kinase activity, usually inactive.

4. Clustering of the receptor brings the kinases in close proximity to start a cross-phosphorylation between receptors.
5. Phosphorylation of the kinases causes an allosteric effect to increase activity.
6. Activated kinases then alter other adaptor molecules consisting of linkers, and other enzymes (e.g., kinases, phosphatases, phospholipases, nucleotide cyclases, and ion channels). The complexes are assembled as a series of scaffoldings resulting in a signal transduction unit.

RECEPTOR ARCHITECTURE AND FUNDAMENTAL CHARACTERISTICS (FIGURE 8.1A–D)

A. Heptahelical receptors
1. Coupled to heterotrimeric G-proteins.
2. Regulates cyclic AMP levels and mediates chemokine activity.
3. Chemokines (chemotaxis, growth and motility).
4. Examples are IL-8, MCP and RANTES.

B. Receptor tyrosine kinase
1. Protein kinase activity is integral to receptor structure
2. Receptor dimerization activates kinase activity, which regulates growth and differentiation
3. Examples are growth hormone, platelet-derived growth factor and insulin.

C. Cytokine receptors
1. Receptor dimerization or trimerization recruits and activates protein kinase activity.
2. Regulates growth and differentiation.
3. Type I receptors respond to most cytokines (Table 8.1).
   a. Signal transducer subunit defines a subset of receptor families.
   b. Binding specificity for a particular cytokine is defined by the receptor subunit.
   c. Redundancy of cytokine activity is due to an exchange of a common signal transducer with the receptor.
   d. Examples are IL-1, IL-2, IL-4 and IL-6.
4. Type II cytokine receptors (Table 8.2)
   a. Receptor and signal transducer activities are found on the same subunit
   b. A second protein with unknown activity is required for functional ligand induced signal transduction.
   c. Three subtypes are known.
      (1) Interferon α/β
      (2) Interferon γ
      (3) IL-10

D. Phosphatase receptors
1. Regulate activation by altering the extent of protein phosphorylation on tyrosine or serine/threonine groups. The phosphatase reverses the effects of kinase activity.
2. Phosphorylation of tyrosine induces the oligomerization of large protein complexes, or scaffolding, which results in very specific signal transduction activities.
3. Regulation of Src kinase activity.
   a. Src kinases have a conserved motif consisting of five modules:
      (1) A tyrosine kinase activity at the C-terminus
      (2) Two domains, SH2 and SH3, are important for folding
      (3) A unique domain-defining structure
      (4) A lipid tail to tether the kinase to the membrane

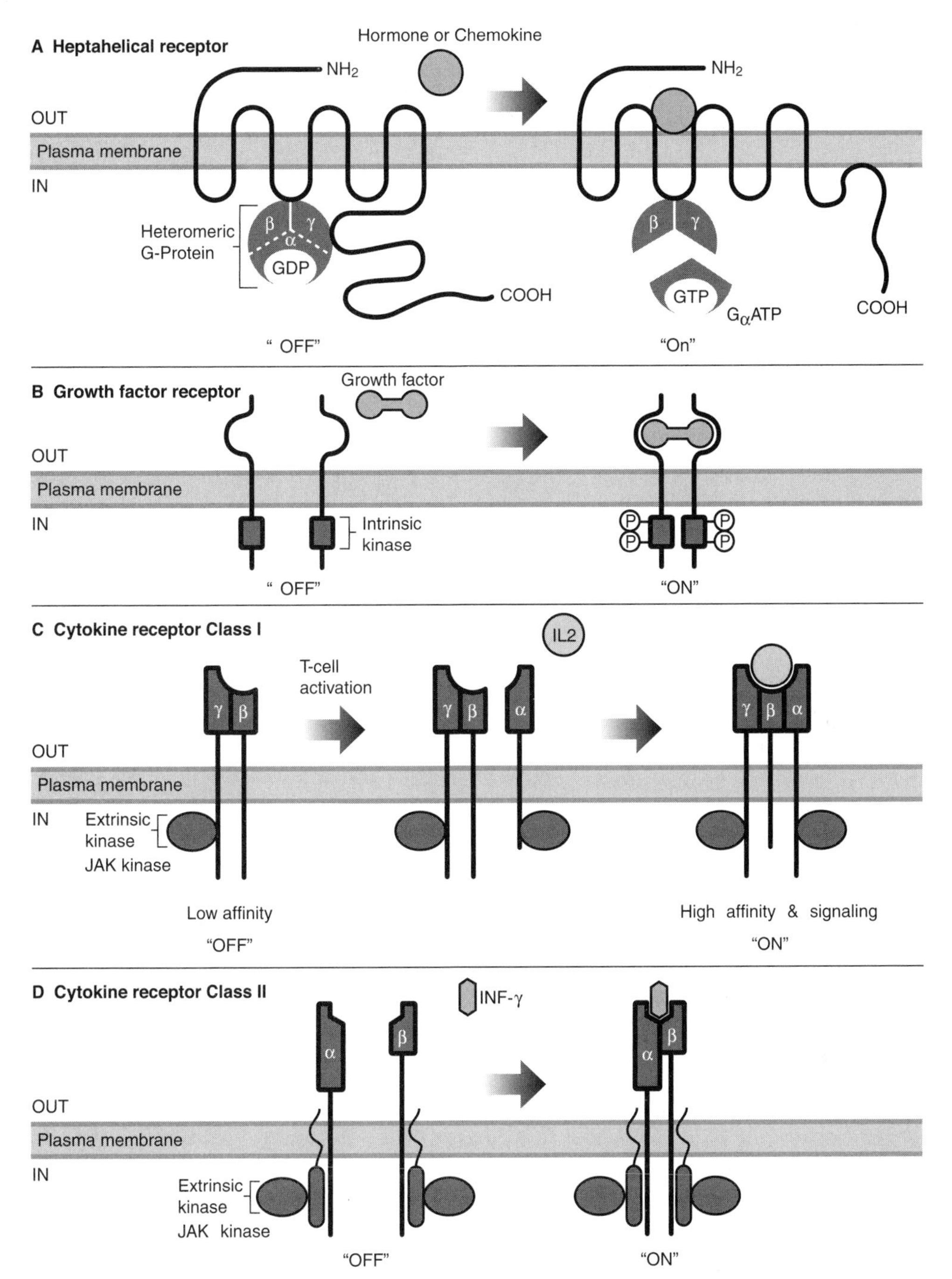

● **Figure 8.1** Receptor architecture of some common signaling systems. *(A)* Heptahelical receptors loop through the plasma membrane seven times and are oriented with the amino terminus to the extracellular side. A heterotrimeric protein complex or G-proteins associates with the receptor in the off state. In the presence of ligand the G-protein complex catalyzes the exchange of GTP for GDP, thereby dissociating a Gα-GTP from the dimeric Gβγ, which both dissociate from the receptor. *(B)* Growth factor receptors associate in the presence of a bivalent ligand to form a dimeric receptor. The cytosolic tail has a kinase activity, receptor dimerization causes a cross-phosphorylation that enhances kinase activity and forms phosphoryl groups for assembling scaffolding. *(C)* Cytokine receptor Class I associate in the presence of ligand to form oligomeric receptors. These receptors form complexes with a separate kinase (Janus Kinase, JAK). The oligmer receptor-JAK complex phosphorylates a cytosolic protein STAT. Each STAT molecule has a SH2 domain such that following phosphorylation by JAK the STAT dimerizes for form an activated transcription factor. *(D)* Cytokine receptor Class II associate in the presence of ligand and a third integral protein to form oligomeric receptors. These receptors form complexes with a separate kinase (Janus Kinase, JAK). The oligmer receptor-JAK complex phosphorylates a cytosolic protein STAT. Each STAT molecule has a SH2 domain such that following phosphorylation by JAK the STAT dimerizes for form an activated transcription factor.

TABLE 8.1 COMPONENTS OF TYPE I CYTOKINE RECEPTORS AND SIGNAL TRANSDUCTION

Signal Transducer (Receptor Subset Family)	Cytokine Receptor Subunit	Non-Receptor Protein-Tyrosine Kinase (JAK[2])	Transcription Factor (STAT[3])
gp130	IL-6 and IL-11	JAK1, JAK2, TYK2	STAT1, STAT3
βc[1]	IL-3, IL-5 and GM-CSF	JAK1, JAK2	STAT5
γc	IL-2, IL-4, IL-7, IL-9 and IL-15	JAK1, JAK3	STAT5

1, common chain; 2, Janus Kinase; 3, signal transducers and activators of transcription.

TABLE 8.2 COMPONENTS OF TYPE II CYTOKINE RECEPTORS AND SIGNAL TRANSDUCTION

Receptor Subset	Non-Receptor Protein-Tyrosine Kinase	Transcription Factor
Interferon α/β (Type I Interferons)	JAK1, Tyk2	STAT1, STAT2, STAT3
Interferon γ (Type II Interferons)	JAK1, JAK2	STAT1, STAT3
IL-10	JAK1, Tyk2	STAT1

b. Src kinases are regulated by a balance between a phosphorylated and non-phosphorylated state.
   (1) Kinase activity is allosterically stimulated by phosphorylation at a tyrosine within the kinase activity module.
   (2) A regulatory tyrosine group located at the C-terminus is the substrate for both kinase and phosphatase activity.
   (3) When the regulatory tyrosine is phosphorylated, the Src kinase folds to sterically block other kinases from gaining access to the allosteric modulating tyrosine; thus, the Src kinase is turned off.
   (4) When a phosphatase removes the phosphate from the regulatory tyrosine, the Src kinase unfolds to reveal the modulatory tyrosine. This intermediary state of unfolding is permissive to activation by other kinase activity. Once unfolded and phosphorylated at the modulatory tyrosine, the Src kinase is turned on.

4. Scaffolding is assembled using phosphorylated proteins as modules to assemble a signal transducing unit.
   a. Phosphotyrosine docks to SH2 groups, specific protein domains found on signaling proteins. Conserved sequence motifs with homology to sequences originally found in the Src oncogene are referred to as SH groups (Figure 8.2).
   b. The SH2 groups work cooperatively with SH3 groups, which bind polyproline sequences, to induce protein conformation changes.
   c. These conformational changes can be used to either activate or inhibit enzymatic activity, or to block or reveal additional docking sites to alter scaffolding.

5. CD45 is
   a. The leukocyte common antigen found on most hematopoietic cells.
   b. Activated by docking between two leukocytes with the phosphatase activity recruited to the region of the dock.
   c. Important for elevating lymphocyte activation response by increasing kinase activities.

6. Calcineurin is a phosphatase used to regulate the activation of the transcription factor NF-AT (nuclear factor–activating transcription).

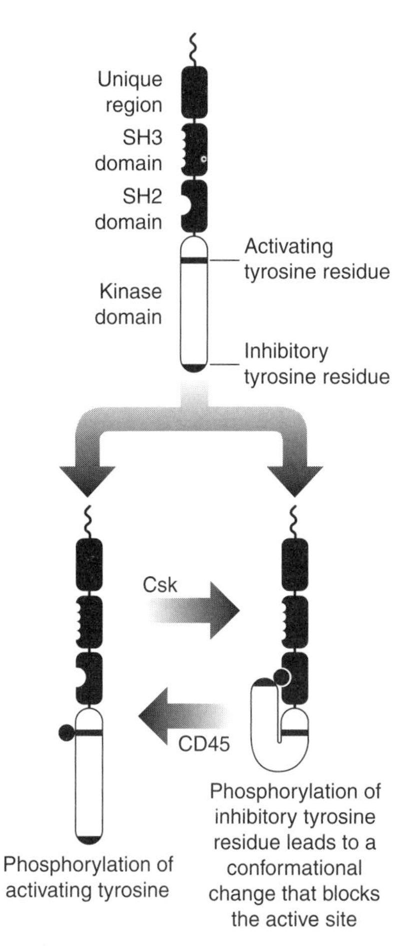

● **Figure 8.2** Regulation of Src-family kinase activity. (Modified with permission from Janeway CA, Travers P, Walport M, Shlomchik MJ: Immunobiology, 5th ed. NY: Garland Publishing, 2001, p 198.) Src-family kinases typically contain two target tyrosine residues for regulatory-kinase activity. Phosphorylation of the inhibitory tyrosine causes a conformational change to block function. Simultaneous phosphatase activity at the inhibitory tyrosine and phosphorylation of the activating tyrosine regulates an allosteric type increase in function.

7. Csk is
   a. The C-terminal Src kinase that is constitutively active in quiescent (resting) cells.
   b. A protein tyrosine kinase (PTK).
   c. Responsible for reversing CD45 and calcineurin activities.

E. Integrin receptors are
1. Dimeric integral proteins that form strong adhesions with extracellular matrices (e.g., fibronectin) or cell-adhesion molecules (e.g., ICAMs and NCAMs).
2. On leukocytes targeted for specific tissues and promote diapedesis, growth, and differentiation.
3. Associated with focal adhesion kinases (FAK) that stimulate transcription via MAP kinase pathway.

F. Hematopoietic cell antigen receptors are (Table 8.3).
1. Antigen directed and define specific host immune responses
2. Multichain immune recognition receptors (MIRR)
   a. Antigen is bound by a receptor chain with no enzymatic activity. Variability changes to adapt specifically to antigen by somatic recombination (see Chapters 5 and 9).
   b. Invariant chains that are non-covalently associated with the antigen binding chain express immunoreceptor tyrosine activation motif (ITAM). The canonical amino acid sequence for ITAM is . . . YXX[L/V]X_{6-9}YXX[L/V] . . .

TABLE 8.3 COMPONENTS OF HEMATOPOIETIC CELL ANTIGEN RECEPTORS

Cell Type	Antigen Receptor	Invariant Chains	Src Kinase
T cell	TCR	[γεεδ] and [ςς]	Lck and Fyn
B cell	BCR (surface IgM)	[αβ] and [αβ]	Fyn, Lyn, and Blk
Eosinophil and mast cells	Fcε High affinity for IgE	[βγγ]	?
Macrophage, NK, and other lymphocytes	Fcγ (CD64, CD16) a) CD64 has high affinity for IgG b) CD16 has low affinity for IgG	[ςς] and [γγ]	?

where Y is the target tyrosine for phosphorylation, L is leucine, V is valine, and X is variable.

c. ITAM is a conserved sequence that is targeted for highly specific phosphorylation by Src kinases.

d. ITAMs direct the assembly of signal transduction complexes

3. T-cell receptor

a. Antigen receptor (i.e., TCR) is composed of a heterodimer of α:β or δ:γ.

b. TCR binds to antigen-MHC complexes on APCs. Recognition by the TCR is MHC restricted, i.e., dependent on three factors:

(1) Antigen contact to the binding groove on the TCR

(2) Contact between the TCR and the MHC

(3) The co-receptor (e.g., CD4 restricts to MHC class II, CD8 restricts to MHC class I).

c. The clustering event recruits co-receptors, CD45, and Src kinases to the TCR to form an ad hoc signal transduction unit.

d. **TCR has no catalytic activity**, only recognition.

4. B-cell receptor

a. Antigen receptor (i.e., BCR) is composed of surface IgM possessing a transmembrane domain.

b. BCR binds antigen and begins to cluster. The clustering event recruits co-receptors, CD45, and Src kinases to the BCR forming an ad hoc signal transduction unit.

c. **BCR has no catalytic activity**, only recognition.

III SIGNALING MOLECULES

A. Adenylyl cyclase is an enzyme that catalyzes the formation of cyclic AMP (cAMP) from ATP. This enzyme is an integral protein found at the plasma membrane and is regulated by the formation of Gα-GTP, a product of the activation of a heptahelical receptor. Formation of cAMP can activate other enzymes (e.g., protein kinase A).

B. Calcium channels are regulated portals for calcium to enter the cytosol. These channels are a diverse family of proteins located on the plasma membrane of the endoplasmic reticulum and can be activated by G proteins, membrane potential, or ligand regulated. An increase of cytosolic calcium can activate a variety of enzymes (phosphatidyl inositol phospholipase and protein kinase C) either alone or with a cofactor (i.e., calmodulin).

C. Calmodulin is a small cytosolic protein that regulates enzymatic activity (calmodulin dependent kinase).

D. Transcription factors that regulate cytokine transcription are NF-AT, NF-κB, and AP-1.

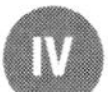

PATHWAYS (examples)

A. Toll-like receptor (TLR) (Figure 8.3)

1. A family of 10 different receptors recognizes PAMP (i.e., viral or bacterial), which stimulates cytokine production (e.g., IL-1, 6, and 12), increased MHC class II expression, and B.7 co-stimulatory signals (e.g., CD80 and CD86). The cytosolic tail of the TLR has structural homology to the IL-1 receptor.

2. Absence of TLR control results in T cell anergy.

3. PAMP binding to TLR stimulates the activation of NF-κB. An example is the signaling initiated by microbial lipopolysaccharide (LPS) binding to the TLR-4.

a. LPS binds to a serum protein called LPS-binding protein, which transfers LPS to CD14. The LPS-CD14 complex then associates with TLR-4 and a third protein called MD2.

b. TLR-4 dimerizes and recruits the adaptor protein MyD88.

c. MyD88 activates a serine/threonine kinase called interleukin-1 receptor associated kinase (IRAK).

d. IRAK activates another adaptor protein called tumor necrosis factor–associated factor 6 (TRAF-6)

e. Oligomerization of TRAF-6 stimulates both the MAP kinase pathway leading to AP-1 activation and the activation of NF-κB.

B. T cell activation (Figure 8.4)

1. TCR-MHC complex begins to recruit adaptor proteins and forms scaffolding.

2. The signal transduction subunits are the CD3 complex and homodimer of ξ (zeta protein).

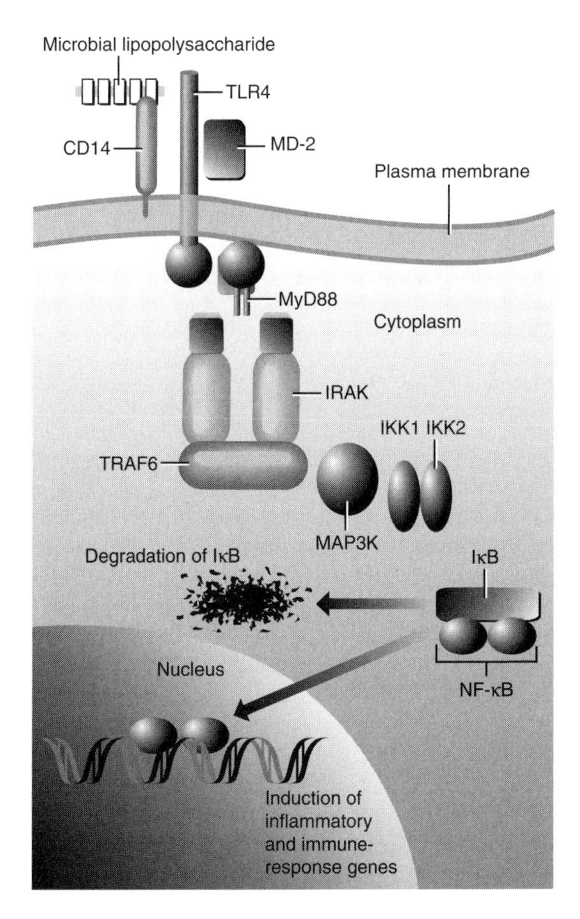

● **Figure 8.3** Signaling pathway of toll-like receptors. (Modified with permission from Medzhitov R, Janeway C Jr. N Engl J Med 2000;343(5):341.) TLR recognize PAMPs to activate antiinflammatory and immune responses. Recognition initiates the activation of NF-κB signaling pathway.

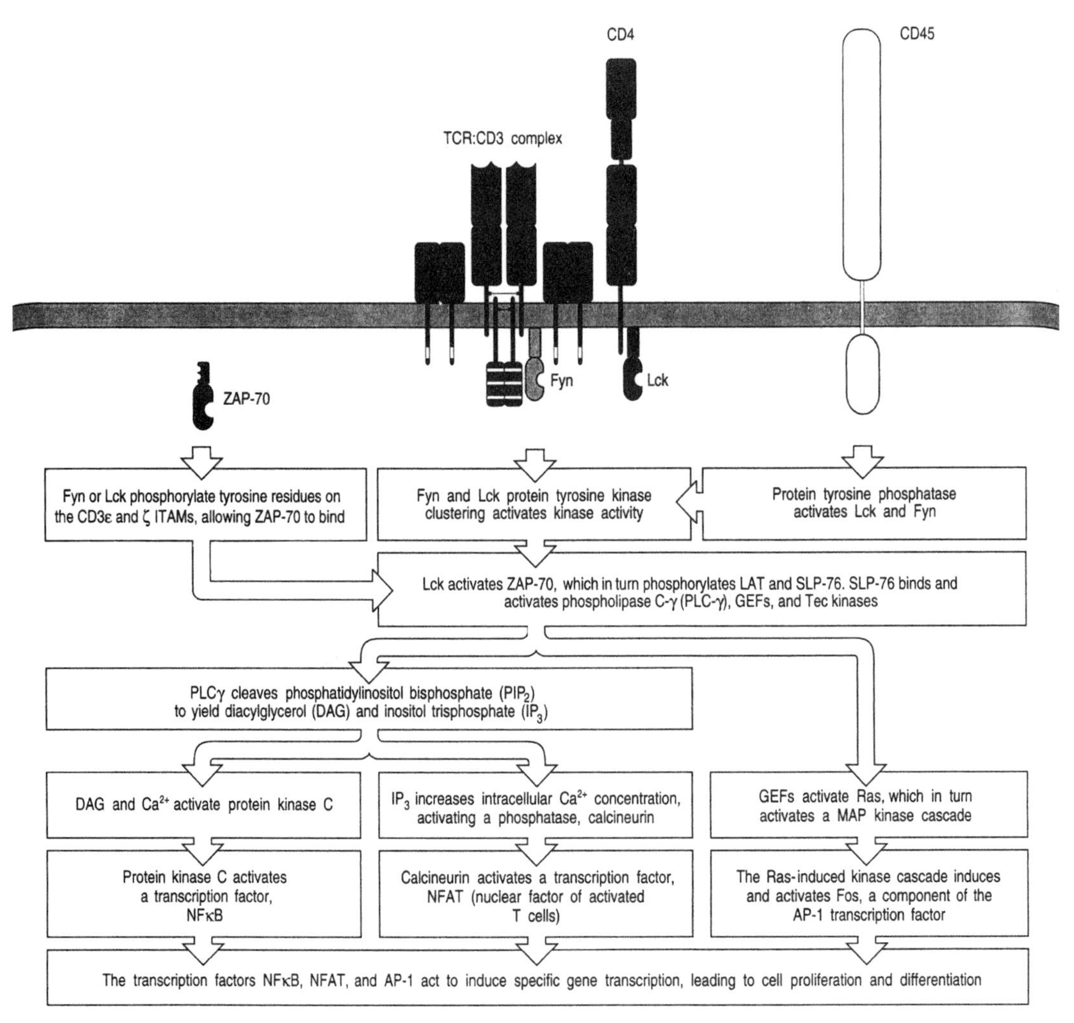

● **Figure 8.4** Peptide-MHC activation of T cells. A co-receptor, CD4, as shown in the figure, binds to MHC class II presented antigen, or CD8 (not shown in the figure) binds to MHC class I presented antigen. The docking of peptide-MHC to the TCR and co-receptor recruits Src kinases to form a cluster that in turn phosphorylates ITAMs found on zeta chains and CD3 molecules. Subsequent building of a scaffold of adaptors and kinases leads to the establishment of signaling complexes that result in phospholipase C activation leading to DAG formation and protein kinase C activation, or activation of small G-proteins. These manifold pathways lead to the activation of the transcription factors NF-κB, NF-AT, and AP-1.

3. Co-receptors CD4 (T_H cells) or CD8 (T_C cells) coordinate TCR docking to peptide-MHC class II or peptide-MHC class I, respectively. The co-receptor is attached to Lck on the cytoplasmic side. Recruiting Lck to the TCR initiates activation by phosphorylating the ITAMs on the zeta chains.
4. Phosphorylated zeta chains form a docking site for the Src kinases ZAP70.
5. ZAP70 is positioned to phosphorylate LAT (linker of activation in T cells). LAT is a cytoplasmic protein tethered to the plasma membrane by multiple palmitate groups. The LAT also has multiple ITAM grouping to allow for multiple dockings with other SH2-containing proteins. Once LAT is phosphorylated the NF-AT, NF-κB and MAP kinase pathway (mitogen-activated pathway) are activated.

C. B cell activation (Figure 8.5)

1. BCR-antigen complex begins to recruit adaptor proteins and forms scaffolding
2. The signal transduction subunits are Igα and Igβ coupled by a disulfide bond. The C-terminus has an ITAM group.

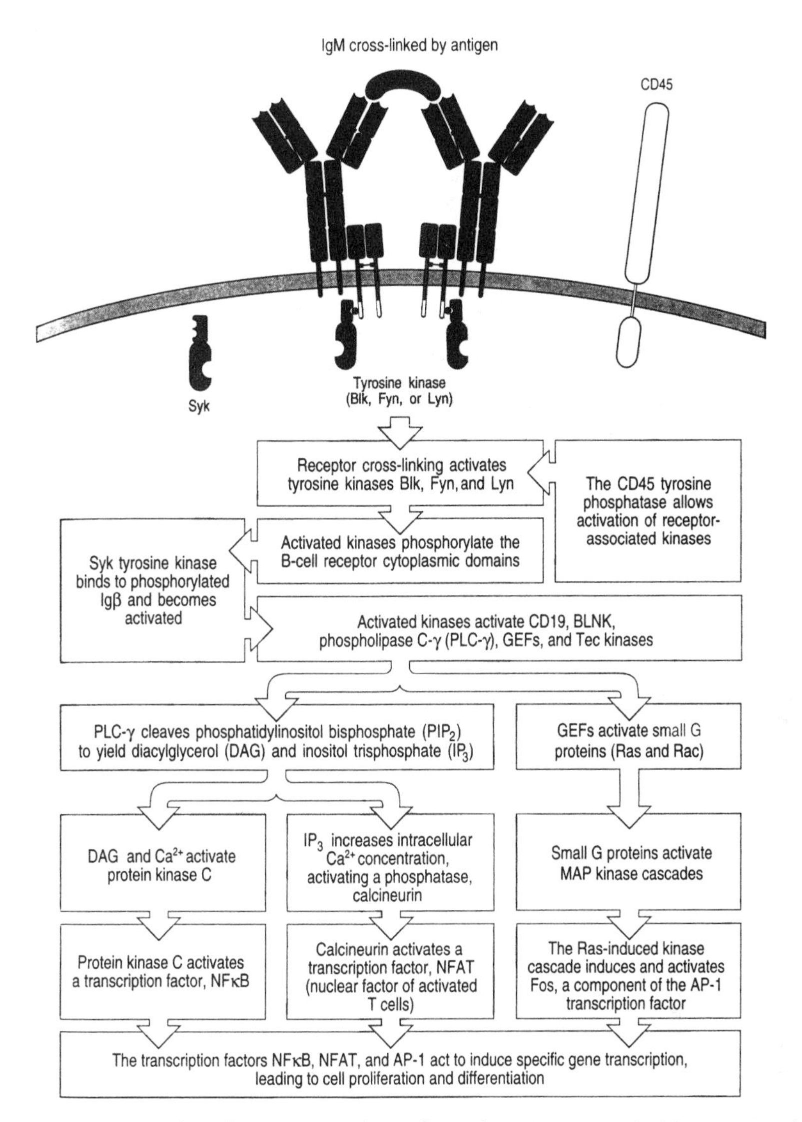

● **Figure 8.5** Antigen activation of B cells. A transmembrane form of IgM is associated with a transmembrane dimer of Igα:Igβ. The IgM binds antigen but cannot signal, the Igα:Igβ signals but cannot bind antigen. Antigen complexing with IgM causes clustering to organize ITAMs found on Igα:Igβ. Src kinases bind to Igα:Igβ to initiate signaling pathways by building scaffolds of adaptor proteins and additional kinase activities. Establishment of the signaling complexes results in Phospholipase C activation leading to DAG formation and Protein Kinase C activation, or activation of small G-proteins. These manifold pathways lead to the activation of the transcription factors NF-κB, NF-AT and AP-1.

3. The co-receptor complex is composed of CD21 (also known as the complement receptor 2 or CR2), CD19, and CD81. Complement C3d fragment can bind CD21 to increase B cell activation by 1000–10,000 fold over only antigen binding to the BCR.
4. Antigen binding to the BCR recruits Src kinases (Blk, Fyn, and Lyn) bound to the Igα:Igβ complex. The clustered Src kinases perform extensive phosphorylation at ITAMs on each other (cross-phosphorylation).
5. Phosphorylated Src kinases become docking sites for Syk, another Src kinase.
6. Syk is positioned to phosphorylate BLNK (B-cell linker protein). BLNK is a cytoplasmic protein tethered to the plasma membrane by multiple palmitate groups. The BLNK also has multiple ITAM groupings to allow for multiple dockings

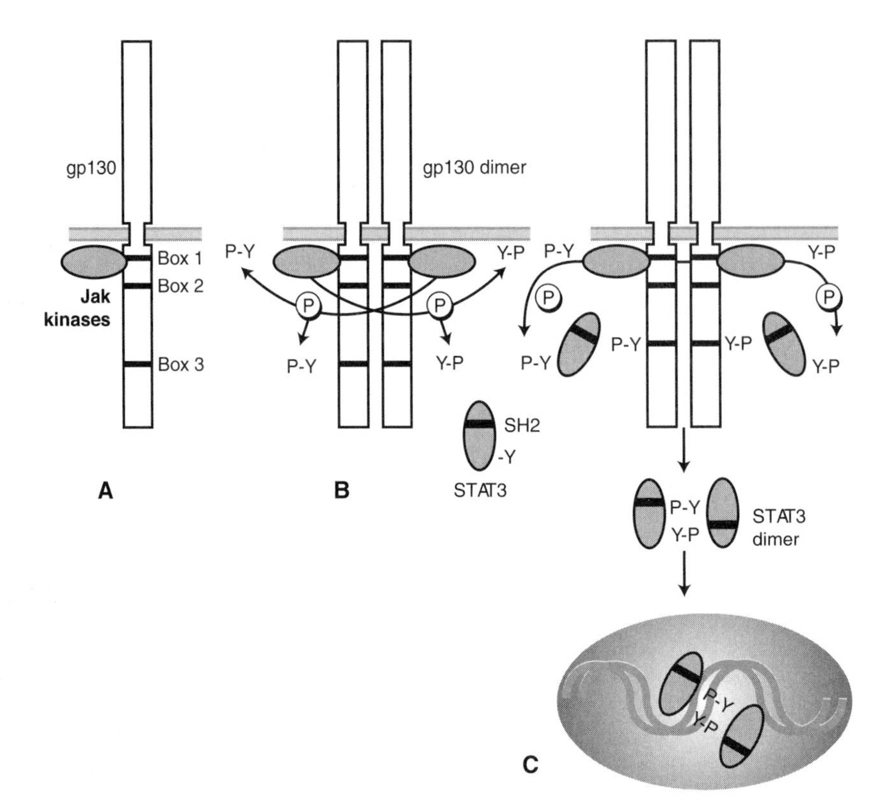

● **Figure 8.6** Interferon γ signaling pathway. (Modified from Heldin CH, Purton M: Signal Transduction. London, Stanley Thornes Ltd, 1998, p 45.) Receptor dimerization leads to JAK activation followed by STAT phosphorylation and dimerization. The STAT dimmer then enters the nucleus to initiate transcription.

with other SH2-containing proteins. Once BLNK is phosphorylated, the NF-AT, NF-κB, and MAP pathways are activated.

D. Interferon-γ (IFN-γ)
   1. IFN-γ is bound by two different receptor subunits.
   2. The formation of a heterologous receptor dimer provides signal specificity.
   3. JAK associated with the receptors phosphorylates STAT.
   4. STAT possesses SH2 domains such that phosphorylated STAT complexes to form dimers. The dimeric STAT is activated and functions as a transcription factor.

E. KAR/KIR
   1. A KAR recognizes host cells and make contact and docks (see Figure 3.2). KAR's docking activates a killing mechanism that initiates cell-mediated killing. The KAR expresses ITAM groups that become phosphorylated and begin assembling adaptor proteins necessary to activate killing activity.
   2. However, a second receptor KIR is available to dock on normal host cells with high levels of MHC class I, an event that blocks KAR activating events. The KIR has an alternate signaling sequence motif called immunoreceptor tyrosine-based inhibitory motif (ITIM). The canonical amino acid sequence for ITAM is . . . [I/V]XYXXL . . . where Y is the target tyrosine for phosphorylation, L is leucine, V is valine, and X is variable. The ITIM groups are also phosphorylated during the KAR activating events. However, phosphorylated ITIM recruits phosphatases (e.g., SHP-1, SHP-2 and SHIP) to the signaling complex. These phosphatases down regulate the KAR activation events by eliminating the phosphorylated ITAM, thus deactivating src kinases.

Chapter 9

Inflammation

INTRODUCTION

A. Definition and cause

1. Inflammation occurs in response to injury resulting from **infection**, **foreign substances** or **other causes**, including antigen–antibody (Ag–Ab) complexes. Inflammation is necessary for **alleviating and repairing injury**; however, excessive inflammation can be **damaging to host tissues.**
2. Inflammation is characterized by the **controlled passage of cells and plasma** from the blood into the traumatized area.

B. Phases. There are two phases of inflammation:

1. **Acute**—mediated primarily by neutrophils
2. **Chronic**—mediated primarily by lymphocytes and macrophages

C. Clinical signs include:

1. **Redness,** caused by increased blood flow, dilation of arterioles, and vascular perfusion of the area
2. **Swelling,** caused by diapedesis of blood cells and plasma from the postcapillary venules into the damaged tissue
3. **Heat,** resulting from swelling and the release of endogenous pyrogens [e.g., interleukin-1 (IL-1), IL-6]
4. **Pain,** caused by the stimulation of neuronal pathways

II INFLAMMATION PROCESS

A. Initiation

1. Inflammation is initiated by the injury-induced release of **pro-inflammatory mediators** (see IV B), including the cytokines IL-1 and tumor necrosis factor-α (TNF-α), as well as complement activated by the alternate pathway.
2. The release of these mediators induces **adhesion molecules** on leukocytes, endothelial cells, and epithelial cells.

B. Recruitment of inflammatory cells into the site by **chemokines** [mainly IL-8 and monocyte chemotactic protein (MCP); see IV A] follows.

1. Initially, **neutrophils** are recruited, followed by **monocytes**, **macrophages**, and, in immune-mediated inflammation, **lymphocytes.**
2. Binding of neutrophil **integrins** to **selectins** and **intracellular adhesion molecules (ICAM)** on the vascular endothelium precedes **diapedesis** into the injury site (Figure 9.1).

C. Damage control

1. Removal of the inciting condition or agent occurs via phagocytic cells that are activated by **IL-8**, **macrophage inflammatory protein (MIP)**, and **interferon-γ (IFN-γ).**
2. Phagocytized, membrane-enclosed organisms are destroyed in the phagocytic vacuole by **lysosomal enzymes and hydrogen peroxide (H_2O_2), nitric oxide (NO), and O_2^- anion**, resulting in oxygen-dependent killing.

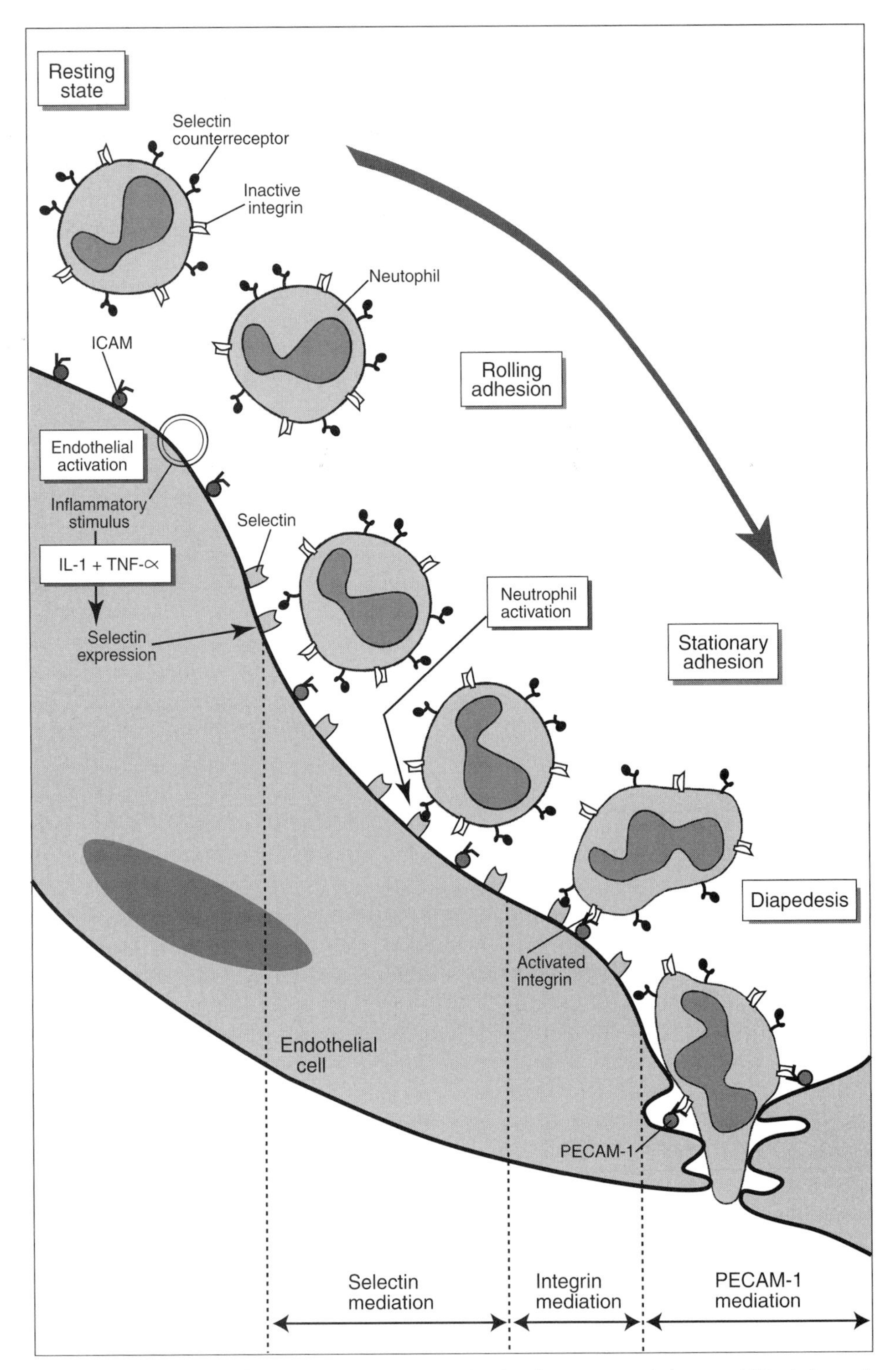

● **Figure 9.1** Following injury and the release of interleukin-1 (IL-1) and tumor necrosis factor-α (TNF-α), the resting state of the endothelium is changed by the appearance of selectins on the cell surface. These selectins bind to the counter-receptor on circulating neutrophils, slowing the polymorphonuclear neutrophils (PMNs) to a "rolling adhesion." The release of IL-8, macrophage inflammatory protein (MIP), and monocyte chemotactic protein (MCP) results in the activation of integrins on the neutrophil surface. The integrins bind tightly to intracellular adhesion molecules *(ICAMs)* on the endothelial cell surface. Diapedesis (transendothelial migration) follows, facilitated by platelet–endothelial cell adhesion molecules *(PECAM-1)*. Antagonism at any point can reduce the inflammatory process. (Modified with permission from Zimmerman GY, McIntyre TM, Prescott SM: Cell adhesion molecules. In *Manual of Vascular Mediators*. Edited by Ward PA. Kalamazoo, MI, The Upjohn Company, 1993.)

D. Repair of the damage caused by excessive inflammation requires two phases.

1. **IL-4, IL-10,** and **transforming growth factor-β (TGF-β)** must **downregulate** IL-8 (a chemokine) and cytokines IL-1 and TNF-α, which initially induced the inflammatory response.
2. **Platelet-derived growth factor (PDGF), TGF-β,** and other growth factors produce an **extracellular matrix** following increased proliferation and activation of fibroblasts.

III KINETICS

KINETICS (see Figure 9.1). Diapedesis is initiated by the slowing and stoppage of the circulating neutrophil.

A. Initiating events

1. Injury-induced, pro-inflammatory molecules activate endothelial cells and trigger the appearance on their membrane of molecules called **selectins.**
   a. **Thrombin** and **histamine** elicit **P-selectin.**
   b. **IL-1** and **TNF** elicit **E-selectin.**
2. Selectins bind loosely to **counterreceptor molecules (L-selectins),** which are present on circulating neutrophils.

B. Rolling adhesion. Binding of the selectin to the counterreceptor slows the neutrophil to a **"rolling adhesion."**

C. Stationary adhesion. Rolling adhesion triggers the activation of integrins [called **leukocyte function–associated antigen-1 (LFA-1)** or CD11a/CD18] on the neutrophil surface. The integrins bind firmly to **intracellular and vascular adhesion molecules (ICAM, VCAM)** after the ICAM and VCAM have been elevated on the endothelium by IL-1, IL-4, and TNF.

D. Diapedesis occurs at intracellular junctions on the endothelium. Migration to the site of injury is facilitated by **chemotactic gradients,** and the cell destruction and later repair begin.

IV MEDIATORS OF INFLAMMATION (TABLE 9.1)

A. Chemokines

1. **Definition.** Chemokines are small-molecular-weight peptides (8,000–16,000 daltons) that are released by injury. These peptides are active at very low concentrations (10^{-8} – 10^{-11} molar) and exhibit approximately 30%–50% amino acid sequence homology.
2. **Function**
   a. Chemokines activate and attract leukocytes to sites with tissue damage.
   b. Chemokines transmit signals through seven transmembrane, rhodopsin-like receptors.
3. **Classification.** Chemokines are classified into two subcategories based on the sequence of two pairs of the amino acid **cysteine.**
   a. **C-X-C chemokines (α)** have their first two cysteines separated by one amino acid.
      (1) Most attract **neutrophils.**
      (2) The most potent include IL-8, platelet factor 4, and IFN-γ-induced proteins, macrophage activation factors, and IFN-γ inducible protein-10.
   b. **C-C chemokines (β)** have two adjacent cysteine residues.
      (1) Most attract **monocytes and T lymphocytes,** while a few attract **eosinophils, basophils,** and **natural killer (NK) cells.**
      (2) C-C chemokines include the **monocyte chemotactic proteins (MCP),** MIP, and **RANTES (Regulated on Activation, Normal T Expression and Secreted).**

TABLE 9.1 MAJOR INFLAMMATORY AND IMMUNE MODULATORS

Cytokine	Cell Sources	Principal Activities
IL-1	Macrophages Fibroblasts Endothelial cells Others	Upregulates adhesion molecules Activates T cells Induces acute phase reactants Synergizes with TNF-α Endogenous pyrogen
IL-2	T cells	T-cell proliferation
IL-3	T cells Thymic epithelial cells	Colony stimulating factor important in early hematopoiesis
IL-4	Th_2 cells	Inhibits Il-8, Il-1, TNF-α Stimulates growth of B cells Induces IgE synthesis
IL-5	T cells Mast cells	Eosinophil growth and differentiation
IL-6	T cells Macrophages Endothelial cells	T and B cell growth and differentiation, APR and fever
IL-8	Monocytes Endothelial cells Fibroblasts	Neutrophil chemotaxis, adhesion, and angiogenesis
IL-9	T cells	Mast cell directed activation of T_H2 response
IL-10	Th_2 cells	Inhibits IL-8, IL-1, TNF-α, and IFN-γ
IL-12	DC Macrophages	Induces CD4 T_H differentiation into T_H1 cells and NK activation
TNF-α	Macrophages, Th1 cells	Activates macrophages, PMNs, and Tc cells Induces PMN-endothelial cell adhesion Causes sepsis, cachexia, pyrexia, acute phase proteins Tumor cell lysis
GM-CSF	T cells Macrophages	Stimulates myelomonocytic cell growth and differentiation into DC
Monocyte chemotactic protein	Endothelial cells Fibroblasts Smooth muscle cells	Induces monocyte, T cell and NK cell chemotaxis Activates macrophages
Macrophage inflammatory protein (MIP)	Macrophages	Activates neutrophil integrins and adhesion to ICAM
Adhesion molecules		
ICAM-1	Endothelial cells	Binds leukocyte integrins to vascular endothelium (same for all adhesion molecules)
ICAM-2	Endothelial cells	
E-selectin (ELAM-1)	Endothelial cells	
VCAM-1	Endothelial cells	
L-selectin (LECAM-1)	Neutrophils	
P-selectin	Platelets, endothelial cells	
LFA (CD11/CD18 integrins)	Leukocytes	Binds neutrophils, monocytes, and lymphocytes to vascular endothelium via ICAMs

TABLE 9.1 MAJOR INFLAMMATORY AND IMMUNE MODULATORS (*continued*)

Cytokine	Cell Sources	Principal Activities
IFN-γ	TH_1 cells NK cells	Induces class I and II MHC Stimulates differentiation of monocytes into macrophages Activates macrophages Inhibits TH_2 cytokines
Soluble IL-2 receptor (sIL-2R)	Enzymatic cleavage of IL-2	Blocks binding of IL-2 to IL-2R High levels in chronic T cell activation
IL-1 receptor antagonist protein	Monocyte secretion	Blocks binding of IL-1 to its receptor
Transforming growth factor-β (TGF-β)	Monocytes, T cells	Induces synthesis of extracellular matrix proteins Assists in wound healing Immunosuppressant
RANTES	Activated T cells	Monocyte chemotaxis
$C^1 5a$	Complement source	Neutrophil chemotaxis and activation Increased capillary permeability

B. Cytokines

1. **Definition.** Cytokines are **intracellular signaling proteins** acting in a **paracrine** or **autocrine** manner. They usually **act locally** by binding to high affinity receptors.
2. **Function.** Cytokines have frequently overlapping functions.
   a. A single activity can be caused by multiple cytokines.
   b. Multiple activities (pleiotropism) can be caused by a single cytokine.
3. **Classification**
   a. **Lymphokines** are cytokines that are produced by lymphocytes.
   b. **Monokines** are cytokines that are produced by monocytes or macrophages.
   c. The cytokine receptors can have **circulating forms**, consisting of only the extra-cytoplasmic portion of the receptor that combines with and blocks the cytokine before it reaches its cellular target (sIL-2R).
4. **Examples** of cytokines include:
   a. **IL-1, IL-6,** and **TNF-α.** These cytokines:
      (1) Induce the acute phase response
      (2) Are endogenous pyrogens
      (3) Induce MCP and IL-8
   b. **TGF-β.** This cytokine:
      (1) Acts as a potent wound-healing agent
      (2) Acts as a potent immunosuppressive agent, inhibiting IL-2 effects and proliferation of many cell types
      (3) Promotes the switching of B cells to immunoglobulin A (IgA) synthesis
5. Cytokine pathways in regulating T helper cells (Figure 9.2)

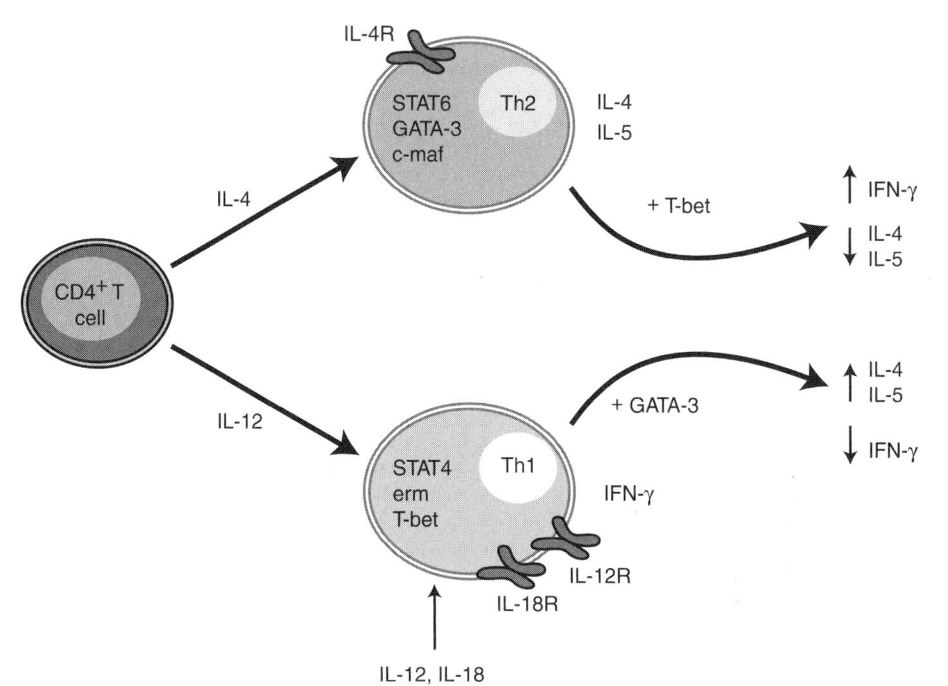

● **Figure 9.2** Cytokine regulation of T helper cell responses. Cytokine IL-12 guides T helper cell development into a Th1 phenotype to initiate cell-mediated immune responses. Cytokine IL-4 guides T helper cell development into a Th2 phenotype to initiate humoral immune responses. Modified with permission from O'Garra A, Arai N. The molecular basis of T helper 1 and T helper 2 cell differentiation. Trends Cell Biol 2000;10:544.

Chapter 10

Hypersensitivity Diseases

I **OVERVIEW.** There are four types of hypersensitivity reactions (Table 10.1).

II **ANAPHYLAXIS (TYPE I) REACTIONS** are termed **immediate hypersensitivity** because symptoms usually begin within minutes in previously sensitized individuals.

A. General characteristics

1. **Classification.** There are two categories of type I reactions:
   a. **Atopy** (local)
   b. **Anaphylactic shock** (systemic)
2. **Definition.** Anaphylaxis is a hypersensitive response by **genetically susceptible individuals** to extremely small amounts of antigen (i.e., **allergen**) to which they already have been sensitized.
3. **Pathogenesis**
   a. **Sensitization** occurs during an initial or repeated exposure to antigens by inhalation, ingestion, injection, or insect sting.
      (1) **Excess IgE antibody** is produced and binds avidly via its Fc domain to its receptor (**FcϵR**) on the surface of **mast cells** and **basophils.** Although a hereditary predisposition to sensitization exists, the IgE antibody does not cross the placenta.
      (2) The **F(ab′)2** containing the antigen-binding sites remains free to bind the allergen.
   b. **Reaction**
      (1) When antigen is **reintroduced** into the **sensitized host**, it binds to and aggregates several cell-bound IgE antibody molecules.
      (2) The resulting membrane perturbation causes **degranulation of the mast cells** and release of pharmacologically active agents (e.g., histamine, leukotrienes, serotonin, bradykinin).
      (3) These agents **rapidly contract smooth muscle, increase vascular permeability and secretions, change coagulability**, and **induce hypotension.**
   c. **Signs and symptoms.** The location of target cells (i.e., mast cells or basophils) determines the resulting signs and symptoms.
      (1) **Mast cells** are abundant in the **skin**, **lungs**, and **mucosae** and do not circulate.
      (2) **Basophils** occur in the **circulation but can be recruited into the tissues.**
4. **Common allergens** include:
   a. Penicillin (active metabolite is penicilloyl)
   b. Procaine
   c. Insect venom

TABLE 10.1 HYPERSENSITIVITY CLASSIFICATIONS

Type	Conditions	Distinguishing Characteristics
I: Anaphylaxis	Atopy Urticaria Asthma Allergic rhinitis Anaphylactic shock	IgE Fc adherence to mast cells and basophils Degranulation and histamine release Smooth muscle contraction
II: Cell surface	Hemolytic disease of the newborn	Exogenous cell antigens
Ag–Ab cytotoxicity	Transfusion reactions	Complement-induced target cell lysis Phagocytosis ABO, Rh blood cell destruction
	Goodpasture's syndrome Glomerulonephritis	Endogenous cell antigens Autoimmunity Complement-mediated neutrophil influx and damage
III: Ag–Ab complex disease	Arthus reaction Serum sickness Polyarteritis nodosa Glomerulonephritis Systemic lupus erythematosus Rheumatoid arthritis	Precipitating antibody Vasculitis Complement-mediated neutrophil influx and damage dsDNA–anti-dsDNA complexes Rheumatoid factor
IV: Delayed-type hypersensitivity	Tuberculosis Granulomatous reactions Contact dermatitis	Cell-mediated immunity Activated macrophages Epithelioid cells TDTH, Th1, CD8+ cells Haptens

Ag–Ab = antigen–antibody; CD = cluster of differentiation; dsDNA = double-stranded DNA; TDTH = delayed-type hypersensitivity effector cells; Th1 = T helper cell type 1.

d. Pollens
e. Molds
f. Foreign serum

B. Atopic disease

1. **Urticaria (hives), a cutaneous form** of immediate hypersensitivity, is characterized by vasodilatation and increased vascular permeability of the skin.
   a. **Incidence.** Urticaria affects approximately 15%–20% of the United States population.
   b. **Pathogenesis. Histamine release** is mainly responsible for the wheal and flare lesion and pruritus.
2. **Asthma** is characterized by **airway obstruction** resulting in acute respiratory distress.
   a. Types
      (1) **Extrinsic asthma** results from **chronic exposure** to occupational, environmental, and food allergens.
      (2) **Intrinsic asthma** can be induced by nonimmunologic means.
   b. Pathogenesis
      (1) **Inflammation** results from the influx of **mast cells, CD4+ cells, Th2 cells, basophils,** and **eosinophils.**

(2) **Obstruction** is caused by **mucus secretion** and mediator-induced **constriction of the smooth muscle surrounding the bronchioles** following allergen–IgE union.

(a) **Important mediators** are the leukotrienes, platelet-activating factor (PAF), eosinophil chemotactic factor (ECF), and histamine.

(b) **Important triggers** are respiratory infections, environmental pollutants, aspirin, nonsteroidal anti-inflammatory drugs (NSAIDs), and isocyanate inhalants.

c. **Signs and symptoms** include wheezing, dyspnea, chest tightness, and cough.

d. **Treatment** includes:

(1) Avoidance of allergen

(2) Drugs that promote bronchial smooth muscle cell relaxation by elevating cyclic adenosine monophosphate (cAMP) [e.g., b-adrenergic bronchodilators, theophylline, aminophylline]

(3) Corticosteroids

(4) Cromolyn sodium

3. **Allergic rhinitis** is the most common clinical expression of atopy.

a. **Clinical features** involve inflammation of the mucous membranes of the nose, leading to profuse rhinorrhea, paroxysmal sneezing, nasal obstruction, itching, and conjunctivitis.

b. **Pathogenesis**

(1) **Common allergens** resulting in allergic rhinitis include pollens, fungal spores, house dust, and animal danders.

(2) **Mediators.** The binding of allergen to cell-bound IgE releases mediators, including histamine, leukotrienes, prostaglandin D_2, and ECF, which attracts eosinophils.

c. **Treatment** is mainly symptomatic. **Desensitization** can be attempted in unresponsive patients.

(1) With certain allergens, a **hyposensitive state** can be achieved by repeated injection of the agent in subliminal doses.

(2) Parenteral exposure to repeated subliminal doses favors the synthesis of circulating **IgG** antibody, which **combines avidly with the allergen in the circulation,** thus **blocking** union with cell-associated IgE and mediator release.

C. **Anaphylactic shock** is a severe, generalized reaction that occurs when the allergen-induced mediators are released **systemically. Anaphylactoid shock** refers to anaphylactic shock induced by nonimmunologic means.

1. **Pathogenesis**

a. **Common triggers** are *Hymenoptera* venom, foods, drugs, and antibiotics (particularly penicillin).

b. **Major mediators** include tumor necrosis factor-α (TNF-α), interleukin-1 (IL-1), IL-6, PAF, leukotrienes, prostaglandins, and histamine.

c. **Death** results from hypotension and shock caused by generalized vasodilation of arterioles, increased vascular permeability, and upper airway edema, leading to organ failure.

2. **Signs and symptoms.** Multiple organs can be affected, leading to symptoms such as hypotension, dyspnea, vomiting, abdominal cramping, angioedema, and urticaria.

3. **Treatment** includes **epinephrine** (which acts as a potent vasopressor), **diphydramine, aminophylline,** and **corticosteroids.**

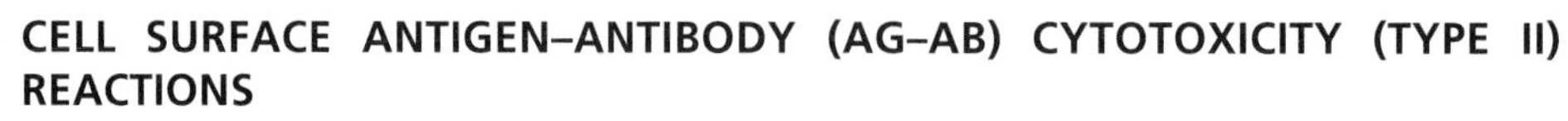

III CELL SURFACE ANTIGEN–ANTIBODY (AG–AB) CYTOTOXICITY (TYPE II) REACTIONS

A. Pathogenesis. Cytotoxicity occurs when antibody is directed against epitopes that occur on the **surface membrane** of host cells. **Damage** results from:

1. **The osmotic, lytic action of complement.** Complement is activated when the antibody binds to the membrane antigen.
2. **Opsonization by phagocytic cells or killing by antibody-dependent cell-mediated cytolysis (ADCC).** Linkage of the Fc receptor and/or the C′3b receptor on the cytotoxic cell to the Fc domain on the antibody bound to the target cell is necessary for ADCC.
3. **Killing of the target cell by cytotoxic T (Tc) lymphocytes, natural killer (NK) cells, or both.** The destruction of the target cell mainly results from the release of perforins and serine proteases (granzymes), which cause pore formation and osmotic lysis.

B. Examples of cytotoxic reactions

1. **Transfusion reactions** occur following the transfusion of blood containing red blood cell (RBC) antigens foreign to the recipient (Table 10.2). **ABO incompatibility** reactions are the most common. **Rh reactions** are the most severe.
   a. Pathogenesis. **Preformed antibodies** in the recipient's blood cause the donor's RBCs to agglutinate, resulting in **complement-mediated RBC lysis** or rapid **phagocytosis.**
   b. Signs and symptoms
      (1) **Fever** is the most common reaction.
      (2) **Chest pain, hypotension,** and **disseminated intravascular coagulation** (DIC) may occur in severe reactions.
2. **Hemolytic disease of the newborn (erythroblastosis fetalis)**
   a. Pathogenesis
      (1) The **major cause** of this disorder is the placental transfer of a non–saline agglutinating, maternal, anti-Rh IgG antibody (usually **anti-RhD**), which binds to RhD+ fetal erythrocytes.
      (2) **Loss of fetal erythrocytes** occurs through complement-mediated lysis or rapid phagocytosis.
         (a) Hemolysis results, causing **hemoglobinuria** and conversion to **indirect bilirubin.**
         (b) The accumulation of indirect bilirubin can result in **respiratory and brain damage.**
         (c) Presence of the antibody in either the mother's circulation or on the infant's cells can be detected by the Coombs tests (of Chapter 6).
   b. **Signs and symptoms** include **hemoglobinuria** and **kernicterus (jaundice).**
   c. **Prevention.** Sensitization of the mother can be prevented by injecting the Rh-negative mother with **anti-Rh antibody** (i.e., **RhoGAM**) within 1–2 days

TABLE 10.2 BLOOD GROUPING

	ABO System			Rh Genotype	
RBC Genotype	**Phenotype**	**Serum Antibody**	**Terminal Epitope**	**Rh+**	**Rh–**
OO	O	Anti-A and Anti-B	Fucose, galactose	DCe	dce
AA or AO	A	Anti-B	N-Acetylgalactosamine	DcE	dCe
BB or BO	B	Anti-A	Galactose	DCE	dcE
AB	AB	Neither	. . .	Dce	dCE

of delivery. This antibody **neutralizes the fetal Rh-positive antigens** entering the mother's circulation during the removal of the placenta, thereby preventing stimulation of the maternal immune system and injury to future Rh-positive newborns.

3. **Autoimmune reactions** occur in **genetically susceptible individuals** who produce antibodies against their own cellular membrane antigens by unknown mechanisms.
   a. **Goodpasture's syndrome** is characterized by **glomerulonephritis** and **pulmonary hemorrhage.**
      (1) The **antigen** is a **glycoprotein** dispersed uniformly on the **glomerular basement membrane (GBM).**
      (2) Susceptible hosts produce an **IgG antibody**, which binds to the membrane antigen and activates complement, releasing the potent chemotactic factor C′5a.
      (3) **Neutrophils** are attracted to the antibody–GBM complex, where they release lysosomal enzymes. These lysosomal enzymes cause **severe necrosis of the glomeruli** and a **loss of filtration capacity.**
   b. **Other autoimmune reactions.** Autoantibodies against many other tissue antigens can occur in the genetically susceptible host and are discussed in Chapter 12.

IV ANTIGEN–ANTIBODY (Ag–Ab) COMPLEX (TYPE III) REACTIONS

A. Pathogenesis. Circulating Ag–Ab complexes of small size, with antigen in slight excess, escape phagocytosis and deposit in tissues or on the surface of blood vessels (Figure 10.1). These complexes can cause damage by:

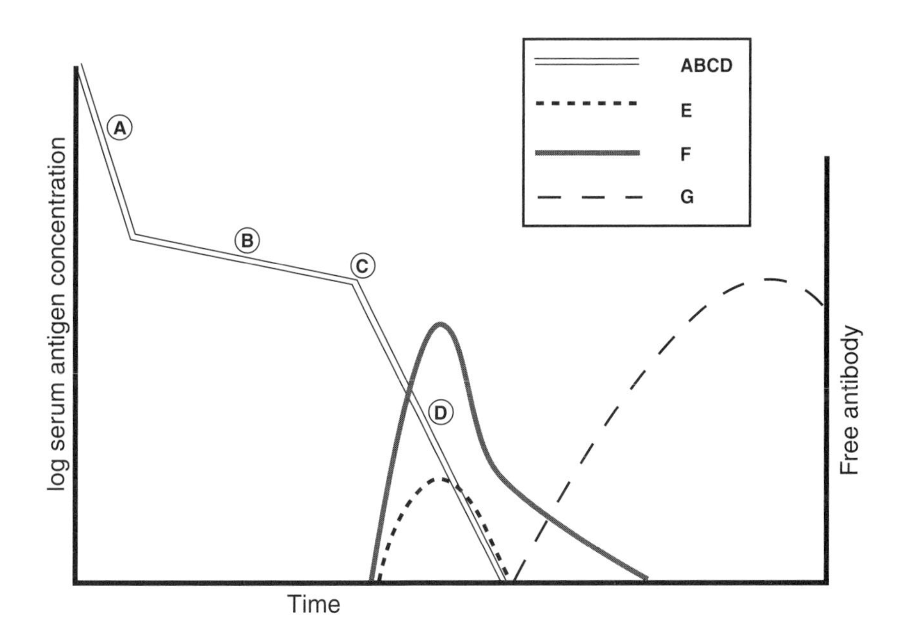

● **Figure 10.1** This graph illustrates the association of pathology (i.e., damage) with the formation of antigen–antibody (Ag–Ab) complexes in an antigen-excess environment. Ag–Ab complex reactions (type III hypersensitivity) result when Ag–Ab complexes, with antigen in slight excess, escape phagocytosis and deposit in the tissues or on the surface of blood vessels. *(A)* Equilibration of antigen between intra- and extravascular spaces. *(B)* Normal serum catabolic phase of antigen. *(C)* Antibody synthesis is initiated; antigen is in considerable excess with a molecular complex ratio of approximately 5:1 (Ag:Ab). *(D)* Rapid disappearance of circulating antigen owing to complex formation with antibody; as antibody synthesis increases, the molecular complex ratio reverses. Curves *E* and *F* describe the appearance of immune complexes (curve *E*) and the interval over which the complexes elicit pathology (curve *F*). Curve *G* describes the later appearance of free antibody in the circulation.

1. **Activating complement and releasing the chemotactic factor C′5a, anaphylatoxins, and clotting factors**
2. **Attracting neutrophils** to the area of deposition, where they release lysosomal enzymes that attack the tissue

B. Examples of Ag–Ab complex reactions

1. **Arthus reaction.** This reaction is a rare, severe inflammatory response to gross, intravascular Ag–Ab precipitates of intermediate size.
   a. The response occurs when **highly sensitized** humans or animals are injected with antigen.
   b. **Complement-activated chemotactic factors** (C′3a, C′5a), **polymorphonuclear neutrophil** (PMN) **infiltration**, and **platelets** result in thrombi and hemorrhagic, necrotic lesions.
2. **Serum sickness**
   a. Etiology
      (1) **Injection of foreign serum** or its products results in a complement-dependent, systemic immune complex reaction.
      (2) A milder allergic vasculitis can be elicited by **drugs** (e.g., sulfonamides, penicillin, cephalosporins, phenytoin, thiourea).
   b. **Signs and symptoms** include fever, a pruritic rash, lymphadenopathy, and joint pain.
   c. **Incidence.** This condition is rare because the use of serum is restricted to the treatment of a few diseases (e.g., hepatitis, tetanus) and immunosuppression.
3. **Polyarteritis nodosa** is characterized by continuous insult of arteriolar walls by the deposition of circulating Ag–Ab complexes, causing **thrombosis** and **obliteration of blood flow.** Frequently, **hepatitis B-antibody complexes** are involved.
4. **Glomerulonephritis**
   a. Pathogenesis
      (1) **Soluble Ag–Ab complexes** (with antigen in excess) deposit on and behind the renal GBM, causing an **inflammatory response.** The release of enzymes by neutrophils attracted to the GBM results in destruction of the glomeruli and loss of filtration capacity.
      (2) The **most commonly implicated antigens** are DNA, insulin, thyroglobulin, group A nephritogenic streptococci, and foreign serum.
   b. **Diagnosis.** Complexes can be detected using **fluorescent antibody** against either the antigen, the antibody, or complement. A **lumpy-bumpy pattern** of fluorescence results from the **random** deposition of the complexes.
5. **Systemic lupus erythematosus (SLE)** is a chronic, exacerbating inflammatory disease that usually affects young women between the ages of 20 and 45 years. The cause of SLE is unknown, but the disorder may be initiated by an antibody response against bacterial or viral DNA, followed by loss of regulatory control of self tolerance.
   a. **Pathogenesis.** SLE is characterized by the **formation of autoantibodies** to many endogenous antigens, such as RBCs, white blood cells (WBCs), platelets, double-stranded RNA (dsRNA), and nuclear antigens [e.g., antinuclear antibodies (ANA)], with **anti-dsDNA** predominating.
      (1) **dsDNA–anti-dsDNA** and other complexes in slight antigen excess randomly lodge in the kidney, giving rise to the **cardinal lesion of glomerulonephritis.**
      (2) **Inflammation** is mediated by a C′5a-induced influx of neutrophils, which results in lysosomal enzyme damage.

b. **Signs and symptoms.** Clinical manifestations of SLE include mainly **polyarthralgia** or **arthritis.** An **ultraviolet light–induced skin rash, facial "butterfly rash," pleurisy, pericarditis,** or **vasculitis** may also be present.

c. **Diagnosis**

(1) A **lumpy-bumpy pattern** of fluorescence distinguishes SLE glomerulonephritis from the Goodpasture type of glomerulonephritis, which is characterized by a smooth pattern.

(2) The **LE cell** (i.e., a neutrophil or macrophage with a phagocytized nucleus), although pathognomonic for SLE, is rarely sought because the technique is cumbersome.

(3) **Rheumatoid factor** may be present.

6. **Rheumatoid arthritis** is a chronic, recurrent inflammatory disease thought to be initiated by an unknown antigen that stimulates local antibody formation in the synovium. Approximately 70% of patients with rheumatoid arthritis possess the **HLA-DR4 haplotype.**

a. **Pathogenesis**

(1) The **union of antigen and antibody** alters the tertiary structure of the antibody, revealing previously buried amino acid sequences "foreign" to the immune system.

(2) These **newly available epitopes** stimulate the local production of an antibody (usually IgM), called **rheumatoid factor.** This antibody can react with the Fc domain of IgG molecules (i.e., an antibody against an antibody). Consequently, IgM–IgG complexes form in synovial fluid and activate complement and chemokines.

(a) **Neutrophils** are attracted to the site. While attempting to phagocytize the complexes, the neutrophils release lysosomal enzymes, destroying articular cartilage.

(b) **Delayed-type hypersensitivity effector** (TDTH) cells predominate and contribute to the damage. Also causing damage are **macrophages,** which release IL-1, IL-6, and TNF, and **osteoclasts,** which injure bone.

(3) **Inflammation** of the pannus and **loss of cartilage** characterize the joint lesions.

b. **Diagnosis.** Rheumatoid factor can be detected by **latex agglutination tests,** which involve the addition of slightly altered IgG-coated latex particles to the patient's serum.

c. Rheumatoid arthritis can also be classified as an autoimmune disease (see p. 73).

V DELAYED-TYPE HYPERSENSITIVITY (TYPE IV) REACTIONS.

The pathologic consequences of cell-mediated immunity (CMI) are referred to as delayed-type hypersensitivity (DTH) and are described in detail in Chapter 7. Tissue damage results from excessive activation of macrophages by cytokines from CD4+ cells, Th1 cells, and CD8+ cells.

Chapter 11

Immunodeficiency Diseases

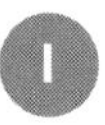

OVERVIEW

A. Disease course

1. **Developmental immunodeficiency disorders** manifest during the **prenatal period** or **early childhood.**
2. A **depressed immune response** also is associated with the **aging process.**

B. Clinical signs include:

1. **A history of recurrent infections**
2. **Below-normal enzyme-linked immunosorbent assay (ELISA)** values for **IgG, IgM,** and/or **IgA** [normal levels, in mg%, are IgG = 800–1400; IgM = 60–200; IgA = 100–300]
3. **Abnormal T cell:B cell ratios, CD4:CD8 ratios,** or **both**
   a. **T cells.** Because all T cells possess membrane-bound CD3, they can be counted by adding **fluorescent-labeled, monoclonal anti-CD3 antibody** to a blood or tissue sample.
   b. **B cells** can be quantified by their reactivity with **fluorescent-labeled, monoclonal antibody** against membrane-bound IgM, CD19, or CD20.
   c. **CD4 and CD8. Monoclonal antibodies** against CD4 and CD8 differentiate **T helper (Th)** and **suppressor** subtypes, respectively.
   d. Normal T/B ratio = 2; normal CD4/CD8 ratio = ~2.
4. **Diminished** *in vivo* **humoral immunity, cell-mediated immunity (CMI),** or **both** against standard vaccines [e.g., diphtheria-pertussis-tetanus (DPT)]

II DEVELOPMENTAL IMMUNODEFICIENCY DISORDERS

A. Transient physiologic hypogammaglobulinemia occurs in infants between the ages of approximately 3 and 6 months. Although infants are born with **adult levels of placentally transferred IgG,** a low level of IgG results from:

1. The disappearance of maternal antibody, which has a half-life of 22–28 days
2. The infant's low early rate of synthesis of secretable immunoglobulins

B. Congenital agammaglobulinemia (Bruton's disease) is a sex-linked (male) disorder that affects infants around the ages of 5 and 6 months. These patients have an apparently normal thymus and CMI.

1. **Clinical features** include:
   a. Recurrent pyogenic infections
   b. Digestive tract disorders
2. **Cause.** The defect that causes Bruton's disease may occur in the transition from pre-B to B cells in the bone marrow and involves the loss of a tyrosine kinase gene. The pre-B cells are normal.
3. **Diagnosis** is made by noting the **absence of tonsils** (on physical examination), **germinal centers** (on lymph node biopsy), and **B cells** (on a peripheral blood smear). **Serum immunoglobulin levels** of less than 10% also suggest the disease.

4. **Treatment.** Passive transfer of **adult serum immunoglobulin** can be administered prophylactically to diminish infections.

C. **Dysgammaglobulinemia.** Patients of varying age present with a **selective immunoglobulin class deficiency** (i.e., one or more immunoglobulins, but not all).

1. **Diagnosis.** Most patients have decreased IgA levels, with 1 in 600–800 individuals affected. Of these patients, many have IgA levels of less than 5 mg/dl compared with a normal value of 300 mg/dl.
2. **Immunologic features** include:
   a. Loss of mucosal surface protection
   b. Failure of IgA-bearing cells to differentiate into secreting plasma cells, although their numbers are normal
   c. Increased susceptibility to autoimmune diseases

D. **Congenital thymic aplasia (DiGeorge syndrome)** is characterized by a **hypocalcemia, tetany,** and an **absence of T cells.**

1. **Cause.** DiGeorge syndrome is **not hereditary.** It is caused by an **unknown intrauterine injury** to the third and fourth pharyngeal pouches that occurs around the **twelfth week of gestation.**
2. **Clinical features**
   a. The **thymus** and **parathyroid glands** are **not developed.**
   b. **Depressed CMI** permits infections caused by opportunistic organisms (e.g., *Candida, Pneumocystis,* viruses).
   c. Patients have apparently **normal germinal centers, plasma cells,** and **serum immunoglobulin.**
   d. Recovery may occur in some patients possessing thymic fragments.
3. Treatment. These patients usually die early.
   a. **Vaccination** with live vaccines (e.g., measles) is contraindicated.
   b. The **transplantation of fetal thymic tissue** is experimental and may be complicated by a graft-versus-host reaction.

E. **Chronic mucocutaneous candidiasis** is a highly **specific T cell disorder** that is characterized by an **absence of immunity to *Candida.*** Patients have apparently normal T cell and B cell absolute numbers and functions. Approximately 50% of patients with this disorder also have endocrine dysfunctions (e.g., hypothyroidism).

F. **Wiskott-Aldrich syndrome** is a sex-linked (male) disorder occurring mainly in children. The syndrome has three main features: **thrombocytopenia** (manifested by bleeding), **eczema,** and **recurrent infections.** An increased incidence of lymphoreticular malignancies or lymphomas may occur.

1. **Immunologic features** include:
   a. Depressed CMI and a low serum IgM level, but normal IgG and IgA levels
   b. Poor response to bacterial capsular polysaccharide antigens
2. **Cause.** The primary defect is on the short arm of the X chromosome and may result in an absence of specific glycoprotein receptors on T cells and platelets.
3. **Treatment. Bone marrow transplantation** may be effective.

G. **Severe combined immunodeficiency disease (SCID)** is a rare disorder characterized by a **genetic defect in stem cells** that results in the **absence of the thymus gland** and **T and B cells.** Affected children are extremely susceptible to infections and have a very **short life span.**

1. **Immunologic features.** A deficiency in the enzyme **adenosine deaminase (ADA)** occurs in 50% of patients. This deficiency results in the accumulation of **toxic deoxyadenosine triphosphate (DATP),** which inhibits ribonucleotide reductase and prevents DNA synthesis. A mutation in the γ chain of the interleukin-2 (IL-2) receptor gene is found in other patients with SCID.
2. **Treatment. Gene therapy** with the ADA gene is experimental.

H. Chronic granulomatous disease (CGD) results from a genetic defect in the **nicotinamide adenine dinucleotide phosphate (NADPH) oxidase system** in neutrophils. Patients are **susceptible to infections** by age 2 years, especially by organisms of low virulence.

1. **Immunologic features. Neutrophil bactericidal activity** (i.e., respiratory burst) is **defective** because of **depressed NADPH oxidase, superoxide dismutase activity**, and **decreased hydrogen peroxide levels.**
2. **Diagnosis** is based on failure of neutrophils and macrophages to reduce a **nitroblue tetrazolium dye.**
3. **Treatment** with **interferon-γ (IFN-γ)** has been successful.

III ACQUIRED IMMUNODEFICIENCY SYNDROME (AIDS)

A. Cause. AIDS is caused by **human immunodeficiency virus (HIV)**, an immunosuppressive RNA retrovirus that is a member of the Lentivirus (slow virus) family.

1. **Two variants** of HIV exist. Both variants closely resemble the simian immunodeficiency virus harbored by African green monkeys.
   a. **HIV-1**, the predominant variant, currently causes disease only in humans.
   b. **HIV-2**, found mainly in Africa, is more readily transmitted heterosexually than HIV-1.
2. **Genetic structure** (Figure 11.1)
   a. The HIV genome consists of **three major genes:**
      (1) ***env*** codes for the **envelope protein**, gp160, which is cleaved into gp120 and gp41.
      (2) ***gag*** codes for the **core proteins** p24, p17, p9, and p7.
      (3) ***pol*** codes for **enzymes** (i.e., **reverse transcriptase, integrase**, and a **protease**).
   b. **Other regulatory genes** include:
      (1) *tat,* which activates transcription of viral DNA
      (2) *nef,* which helps with virus replication
      (3) *rev,* which regulates mRNA activity

B. Pathogenesis. The **major target cell** is the **CD4+ Th cell,** which is eventually lysed by the virus. Several other cells (e.g., macrophages, astrocytes, dendritic cells) with much lower membrane levels of CD4 can be infected by low numbers of HIV. Because these cells are not readily lysed, they may serve as reservoirs of latent virus.

1. **Virus entry**
   a. HIV can also enter macrophages and/or dendritic cells by binding both to the CD4 receptor and an obligate chemokine coreceptor (CCR5) via gp120.
   b. After the virus binds to the CD4+ Th cell and its obligate chemokine receptor, CXCR4, via gp120, fusion and entry of the virus through the cell membrane is mediated by gp41.
2. **Transcription of the viral RNA into DNA** is accomplished enzymatically through a viral **reverse transcriptase.**
3. **Integration of viral DNA into the target cell** genome is facilitated by an **integrase**, leading to the formation of a **provirus** that may lie latent for years.
4. **Host cell lysis.** Following activation of the infected T cell (by other viruses or antigens), the provirus is transcribed, translated into viral proteins, assembled, and replicated, leading to lysis of the host cell.
5. **Infections and cancer**
   a. **Infections.** Depletion of the Th cell population results in a loss of cytokines (which activate other immunocompetent cells) and a diminished capacity to offset normally noninvasive, infectious agents. Infections in patients with AIDS are caused primarily by **endogenous** and **nosocomial agents.** Common

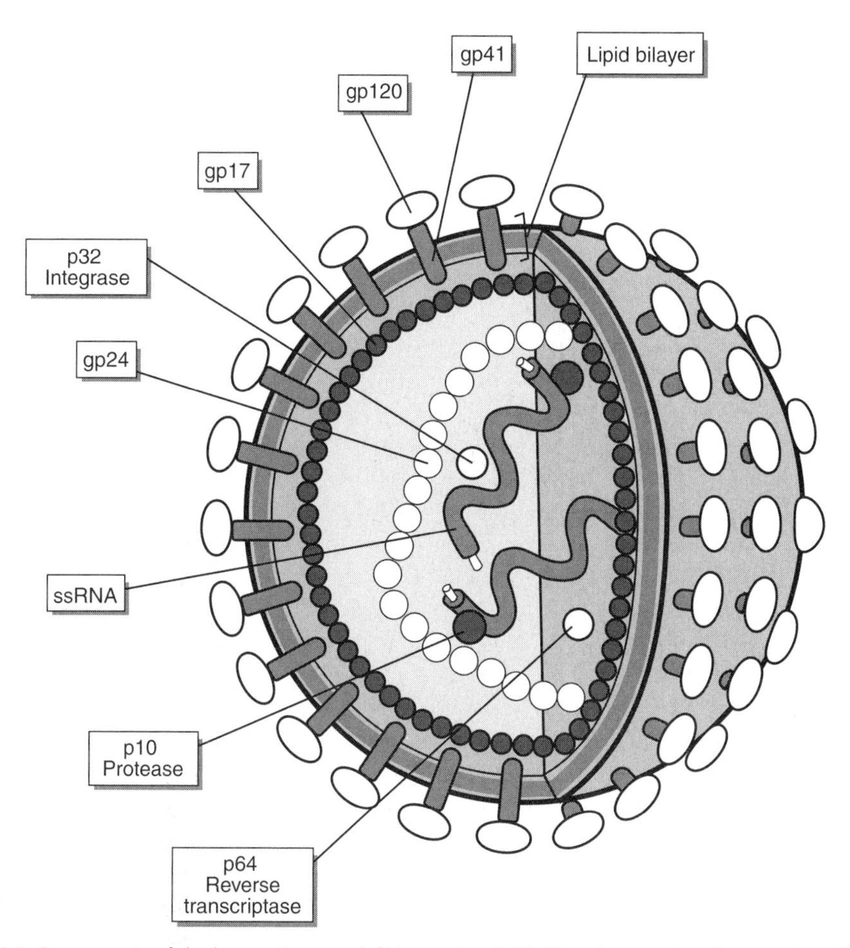

● **Figure 11.1** Components of the human immunodeficiency virus (HIV). The virus consists of an envelope formed from glycoproteins (i.e., gp120 and gp41) that houses several core proteins (e.g., p17, p24). The virus has several genes that code for enzymes (e.g., integrase, reverse transcriptase, protease) that play a role in integrating viral DNA into the host genome and degrading polyprotein precursors into smaller proteins and peptides.

organisms include ***Pneumocystis*, cytomegalovirus** (CMV), ***Toxoplasma*, *Candida*, *Mycobacterium*, herpesvirus**, and ***Cryptococcus***.

(1) At **CD4 T cell levels of 200–400 cells/µl**, ***Candida albicans*, *Mycobacterium avium-intracellulare*,** and **varicella-zoster** infections dominate.

(2) At **CD4 T cell levels of less than 200 cells/µl**, ***Pneumocystis carinii*, CMV**, and ***Cryptococcus neoformans*** are common causes of infection.

b. Cancer

(1) HIV-positive patients are predisposed to **Kaposi's sarcoma** (mediated by herpes simplex virus-8).

(2) There is a markedly increased susceptibility to highly aggressive **B cell lymphomas**, notably **Burkitt's lymphoma** and **immunoblastic sarcoma**, among HIV-positive patients.

C. Diagnosis

1. **Signs and symptoms.** Patients with HIV can present with any number of **vague symptoms** (e.g., fever, weight loss), making clinical diagnosis difficult. One notable clinical sign is **increased frequency of infections by opportunistic organisms.** These infections often occur at relatively predictable CD4+ counts.

2. **Laboratory tests**
   a. **ELISA.** Positive results on two separate tests are suggestive. Indirect ELISA tests detect serum antibody to HIV.
   b. **Western blot.** This test confirms the ELISA tests.
   c. **Polymerase chain reaction (PCR).** If necessary, small amounts of HIV DNA can be amplified using PCR.

D. **Treatment** is based primarily on interference with some stage of the HIV life cycle.
   1. **Reverse transcriptase inhibitors.** Inhibition of reverse transcriptase by the dideoxynucleotides has slowed but not ceased the progression of the disease. Agents include:
      a. Zidovudine (ZDV)
      b. Azidodideoxythymidine (AZT)
      c. Dideoxyinosine (ddI)
      d. Dideoxycytidine (ddC)
   2. **Protease inhibitors** have recently become available. These agents prevent the cleavage of protein precursors, which are essential for HIV maturation.
      a. **Agents. Saquinavir, ritonavir, indinavir,** and **nelfinavir** reduce viral loads when used in various combinations.
      b. **Effectiveness.** None of these protease inhibitors has completely eradicated viral reservoirs, and HIV resistance is beginning to develop.

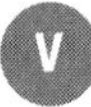

CYTOKINE AND CHEMOKINE DEFICIENCIES. A functional deficiency in any of the 18 cytokines or 40 chemokines described to date, or their receptors, would contribute to an immunocompromised state.

A. **Cytokines** regulate cell–cell signaling.
B. **Chemokines** have chemoattractant properties.
C. **Specific receptors on target cells** control cytokine and chemokine action.

V SENESCENCE (AGING) OF THE IMMUNE RESPONSE

A. **T cells.** Although T cell levels remain in the normal range, there is a loss in some T cell functions in the elderly. This loss results in **depressed humoral and cellular immune responses,** which are highly variable in the aged.
B. **Autoimmune diseases** are more prevalent, suggesting defects in immune regulation.

Chapter **12**

Autoimmune Disorders

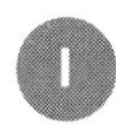

OVERVIEW

A. Definition. Autoimmune disorders result in antibody or cell-mediated immunity (CMI) against the host's own tissues.

B. Immunologic mechanisms

1. **Self-tolerance.** Normally, humans are **immunologically unresponsive to endogenous molecules** because of self-tolerance. However, in normal humans, B-cell clones do exist, with receptors reacting with endogenous molecules (self-antigens).
2. Tolerance to self-antigens can be achieved by **clonal deletion**, **clonal anergy**, or **peripheral suppression**. A breakdown in any of these three mechanisms results in aberrant immunologic regulation and autoimmunity.
   a. **Clonal deletion.** This hypothesis postulates a loss in self-reactive T and B cells, which appear during maturation in the fetal thymus and bone marrow.
      (1) **Immature CD4+ T cells**, which bear receptors for endogenous molecules, are eliminated after contact with self-antigens in the **thymus gland.**
      (2) **Immature B cells with self-reactive receptors** are destroyed after contact with potential self-antigens in the **bone marrow.**
   b. **Clonal anergy** describes the loss of T- and B-cell functions after exposure to antigens in the absence of mandatory costimulatory signals (e.g., B7–CD28 binding), or following exposure to cells lacking major histocompatibility complex (MHC) class II molecules.
   c. **Peripheral suppression** can occur if **CD8+ T cells or macrophages secrete cytokines** [e.g., transforming growth factor-β (TGF-β)], which downregulate the immune response, or if **tolerogenic doses of antigen are administered.**
      (1) **High-dose tolerance** is an anergic condition that occurs after systemic exposure to large amounts of unaggregated proteins.
      (2) **Low-dose tolerance** occurs after repeated administration of small amounts of protein antigens.
      (3) A **tolerant state** also can be induced by certain antigens when administered orally.
      (4) Tolerance is specific, more readily induced, and lasts longer in T cells than in B cells.

II IMMUNOREGULATION BREAKDOWN.

The theories of why immunoregulation breakdown results in autoimmunity vary with the disorder. These theories include:

A. Cross-reaction of microbial antigens with human tissue antigens (molecular mimicry)

1. Although this reaction induces an immune response against the host, this is **not true autoimmunity** because the antigenic stimulus is of **exogenous origin.**
2. **Examples** of this theory include:
   a. **Streptococcal antigens**, which stimulate an immune response that cross-reacts with sarcolemmal heart muscle and the kidney.
   b. **Anti-DNA antibodies** (which may be induced by microbial DNA) that react with cells in patients with **systemic lupus erythematosus (SLE).**
   c. Deposition of **viral antigens** on host-cell membranes in which the immune response against the virus includes damage to the host cell.

B. Sequestration of potential self-antigens from fetal clonal deletion-inducing mechanisms. Antibodies to self-antigens in thyroid and heart tissue emerge after the tissue is **damaged by microbes or surgery.** These antibodies **rarely cause injury.**

C. Formation of new antigenic determinants. The alteration of host molecules exposes the host to new antigenic determinants that were **unavailable when fetal tolerance was induced.** For example, patients with rheumatoid arthritis exhibit **rheumatoid factors**, which are mainly IgM antibodies against the Fc fragment of IgG. The Fc is altered and becomes antigenic when IgG formed in the synovium complexes with an unknown antigen.

D. Formation of a hapten-carrier complex. The adsorption of a foreign hapten (e.g., **quinidine, sulfathiazole**) onto an endogenous molecule (e.g., **platelets**) leads to the formation of a hapten-carrier complex. Antibody to the drug is formed and reacts with the drug on the platelet membrane. Complement is activated, resulting in **platelet lysis.**

E. Depletion of suppressor cells

1. If the normally occurring suppression (by T-suppressor cells) of B-cell clones that arise with idiotype specificity for self-antigens is lost or diminished (as in elderly patients), autoantibodies result.
2. An inordinate **switch from Th1 to Th2 cell activation** during antigenic stimulus may favor **autoantibody synthesis.**

III SYSTEMIC AUTOIMMUNE DISORDERS

A. SLE is an episodic multisystemic disease that usually occurs in young women.

1. **Clinical signs.** An **erythematous rash, vasculitis**, and **arthritis** are the major lesions. In addition, **nephritis** may be seen.
2. **Immunologic features**
   a. SLE is characterized by **multiple autoreactive antibodies** against diverse cellular constituents.
      (1) **Antinuclear antibody (ANA).** The most dominant antibody is ANA, which is nonspecific and may be induced by microbial infection.
      (2) Antibodies to **double-stranded DNA (dsDNA)** are **specific for SLE.**
   b. **Immunologic mechanisms**
      (1) Small **antigen–antibody (Ag–Ab) complexes** with host antigen in excess continuously deposit on and behind the glomerular basement membrane (GBM).
      (2) The accompanying **complement fixation releases C′5a**, which attracts inflammatory cells into the area of complex deposition.
      (3) **Damage.** Subsequent release of leukocytic lysosomal enzymes **damages the GBM** and **impairs renal filtration.**
3. **Differential diagnosis**
   a. SLE can be confused with **rheumatoid arthritis** because 30% of SLE patients exhibit serum rheumatoid factor.

b. **Certain drugs** (e.g., procainamide, hydralazine, quinidine, chlorpromazine) can induce a **lupus-like syndrome.**

B. **Rheumatoid arthritis (RA)** is a chronic, systemic inflammatory disease that is characterized by **granulation tissue (pannus) formation** and **subcutaneous nodules** in the joints.

1. **A genetic predisposition** (HLA-Dw4 and HLA-DR4) for this condition exists.
2. **Immunologic features.** Antibodies against immunoglobulins, called **rheumatoid factors**, appear in serum and synovial fluids. Rheumatoid factor formation may be an **immune response** by synovial lymphocytes **against antibody complexed to an unknown antigen.**
   a. **Complement** is activated, and the resulting chemotactic factors attract inflammatory cells into the joints, which release collagenase.
   b. **Damage.** These inflammatory cells damage tissues by releasing cytokines and pharmacologically active mediators (e.g., PMNs, osteoclasts).
3. **Diagnosis.** Rheumatoid factors in patients serum can be detected by the agglutination of latex particles coated with altered IgG.
4. RA is also classified as a hypersensitivity disorder (see Chapter 10).

C. **Sjögren's syndrome** is a chronic inflammatory disease of **unknown etiology** that primarily affects **postmenopausal women.** This syndrome may occur **secondary to rheumatoid arthritis** and SLE.

1. **Clinical features** include **dryness of the mouth, trachea, bronchi, eyes, nose, vagina,** and **skin.**
2. **Immunologic features.** Sjögren's syndrome is characterized by autoantibodies against salivary duct antigens, lymphocytic infiltration, and immune complex formation in the salivary gland.

D. **Polyarteritis nodosa** is one of several **human vasculitides** of varying cause. The condition often involves hepatitis B Ag–Ab complexes, which are found in the vessel walls of 30%–40% of patients. Similar lesions can be reproduced in animals using other Ag–Ab complexes.

IV ORGAN-SPECIFIC AUTOIMMUNE DISORDERS

A. Blood disorders

1. **Anemia, leukopenia, and thrombocytopenia.** Autoantibodies that react with **red blood cells (RBCs), white blood cells (WBCs),** and **platelets** result in anemia, leukopenia, and thrombocytopenia, respectively.
2. **Multiple myeloma,** the malignant transformation of a single plasma cell clone, as manifested by a single spike on electrophoresis, results in an excess of IgG or another immunoglobulin class **(paraproteins).** Patients may secrete **Bence Jones proteins** (monoclonal light chains) in their urine.

B. Central nervous system (CNS) disorders

1. **Allergic encephalomyelitis** is a demyelinating disease that can occur after infection or immunization.
   a. The condition can be mimicked experimentally by immunizing animals with **homologous extracts of brain** or a **nonapeptide** from the basic protein of myelin.
   b. The experimental disease can be transferred to normal animals with **lymphocytes sensitized to the nonapeptide,** implicating CMI in the demyelination process.
2. **Multiple sclerosis** is a chronic, relapsing disease of unknown etiology that is characterized immunologically by mononuclear cell infiltrates and demyelinating lesions (plaques) in the white matter of the CNS.

a. **Clinical features.** Patients usually have **increased levels of IgG** in the cerebrospinal fluid. Elevated titers to measles and other viruses appear in the cerebrospinal fluid, suggesting a viral etiology.

b. **Immunologic features.** Patients with MS generally exhibit a **decrease in suppressor T-cell function**, which indicates an immunoregulatory disorder.

3. **Myasthenia gravis** results from a defect in neuromuscular transmission.

a. **Clinical features** include **muscle weakness** and **fatigue.** Patients often exhibit **thymic hyperplasia** or a **thymoma.**

b. **Immunologic features**

(1) Myasthenia gravis is associated with the presence of an **anti-acetylcholine receptor antibody.** Binding of this antibody with the receptor at the postsynaptic membrane of the neuromuscular junction results in the loss (**endocytosis**) of the receptor.

(2) An **inability to transmit the acetylcholine-induced signal** to muscle fibers results and causes the clinical signs.

C. Endocrine disorders

1. **Chronic thyroiditis (Hashimoto's disease, hypothyroidism)** is a self-limiting disease with a probable genetic basis that affects mainly women.

a. Chronic thyroiditis is characterized by autoantibodies and CMI to thyroglobulin or thyroid peroxidase. This reactivity causes progressive **destruction of the thyroid gland.**

b. **Antibody-dependent cell-mediated cytotoxicity** (ADCC) may be responsible for the tissue damage.

2. **Graves' disease (hyperthyroidism)** is characterized by T cell and B cell infiltration of the thyroid gland, leading to the formation of **autoantibodies** to the **thyroid-stimulating hormone (TSH) receptor.** The autoantibodies may compete with TSH, bind to the TSH receptor site, and induce uncontrolled TSH-like activity. Clinical features include a diffuse goiter and thyrotoxicosis.

3. **Diabetes mellitus (insulin-dependent diabetes, juvenile onset, type I diabetes)** is characterized by the destruction of insulin-producing cells in the pancreas. Either humoral or cell-mediated anti-islet cell activity can be operative. There is no evidence of an autoimmune pathogenesis for non–insulin-dependent (maturity onset, type II) diabetes.

D. Gastrointestinal tract disorders

1. **Pernicious anemia** is caused by impaired gastrointestinal absorption of vitamin B_{12}, resulting in weakness and chronic fatigue.

a. **Immunologic features**

(1) Pernicious anemia occurs secondary to **T cell damage** to the **gastric parietal cell.** The gastric parietal cell normally synthesizes **intrinsic factor**, the agent responsible for the transport of vitamin B_{12} into the blood.

(2) **Anti-parietal cell** and **anti-intrinsic factor antibodies** are found in most patients. The latter block the transport function of intrinsic factor and contribute to the disease process.

b. **Treatment.** Injection of vitamin B_{12} bypasses the need for gastric absorption and corrects the deficiency.

2. **Ulcerative colitis** is characterized by chronic **inflammatory lesions** that are confined to the **rectum** and **colon.** These lesions are accompanied by the **infiltration of monocytes, lymphocytes,** and **plasma cells.**

a. Patients' lymphocytes exert cytotoxicity against colonic epithelial cells in culture.

b. Patients may also have antibodies that are cross-reactive with ***Escherichia coli***, but the disease is of **unknown etiology**.

3. **Crohn's disease** is an inflammatory, granulomatous disease that involves **T and B cells, macrophages**, and **neutrophils**. The disease usually occurs in the **submucosal area** of the **terminal ileum**. This chronic progressive disease is often suspected but has not been established as being of **microbial etiology**.
4. **Chronic active hepatitis** is characterized by an **infiltration of the liver by CD8+ T cells, B cells**, and **monocytes**. The condition may result from **faulty immunoregulation** because of decreased suppressor cell numbers.

Chapter **13**

Immunologic Aspects of Transplantation

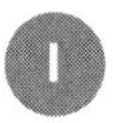

HISTOCOMPATIBILITY. Rejection of transplanted organs and tissues is antigenically specific and is determined primarily by allogeneic differences in the **histocompatibility antigens [i.e., human leukocyte antigens (HLAs)]** between donor and recipient. The genes for the HLAs are located in the major histocompatibility complex (MHC) on chromosome 6.

A. HLA function. HLAs have two functions:

1. Their major **physiologic function** is to **bind and present processed, foreign antigenic peptides** to T cells, thus initiating the immune response (see Chapter 5).
2. They also **distinguish the MHC membrane antigens** on a transplanted donor organ from those of the recipient, provoking an attack by the recipient's sensitized T cells.

B. HLA classification. Class I and class II HLA genes, which encode antigens, exhibit enormous polymorphism, inasmuch as multiple different alleles exist at each locus.

1. **Class I antigens** are found on all **nucleated cells.**
   a. **Structure.** Class I antigens have three gene loci: **HLA-A, HLA-B,** and HLA-C.
   b. **Identification.** These antigens are defined serologically with anti-HLA antibodies.
   c. **Function.** Class I antigens present foreign antigenic peptides to **CD8+ cells.**
2. **Class II antigens** are found on **immunologic effector cells** (e.g., macrophages, dendritic cells, B cells, activated epithelial cells).
   a. **Structure.** Class II antigens have three gene loci within the D region: **HLA-DP, HLA-DQ,** and **HLA-DR.**
   b. **Identification.** These antigens are defined by cellular reactions.
   c. **Function.** Class II antigens present foreign antigenic peptides to **CD4+ cells.**

C. Tests for histocompatibility. Matching the donor and recipient at the HLA locus improves graft acceptance (Table 13-1).

1. Both donor and recipient are typed for **HLA profiles** using DNA sequence analysis of the HLA genes or more than 200 specific anti-HLA antisera.
2. Both donor and recipient are **typed for ABO and Rh antigens** with specific antisera.
3. The donor must be tested for **preexisting anti-HLA antibodies** and **cell-mediated immunity (CMI)** because sensitization to HLA antigens can occur as a result of **prior blood transfusions, pregnancy,** or **other organ grafts.** One way to test for preexisting anti-HLA antibodies and CMI is with a **mixed lymphocyte culture.**
   a. **Procedure**
      (1) **Blood lymphocytes** from the donor and the recipient are cultured together, and **tritiated thymidine** is added.

TABLE 13-1 **TYPES OF GRAFTS**

Type	Condition	Fate
Autograft	Within the confines of one's own self	Accepted
Isograft	Between members of an inbred species	Accepted
Allograft	Between members of a species (humans)	Rejected
Xenograft	Between members of different species	Rejected
Homovital	Viable, functional graft required	. . .
Homeostatic	Nonviable graft, used for support	. . .

(2) The donor cells are treated with an **antimitotic agent**; therefore, any response can be attributed to the recipient's reaction against the donor's cells.

b. **Results**

(1) If the lymphocytes are antigenically incompatible, DNA is synthesized, and the cells divide.

(2) The extent of the genetic disparity can be determined by scintillation counting.

II COMPLICATIONS OF ORGAN TRANSPLANTATION

A. Graft rejection. The vigor and speed of rejection is related to the genetic disparity between the donor and the recipient (i.e., the degree of foreignness). CD8+ cytotoxic T (Tc) cells and macrophages (activated by CD4+ T cells) mediate most rejections.

1. Acute rejection

a. **Definition.** Acute rejection, characterized by swelling and tenderness over the allograft, occurs within weeks. The exact time of onset varies with the host, the organ, and the immunosuppressive regimen.

b. **Mechanism of rejection.** HLA antigens on allografts stimulate recipient CD4+ T cells, which respond by secreting cytokines and by inducing adhesion molecules.

(1) **Interleukin-2 (IL-2)** activates **CD8+ T cells** to a state of cytotoxicity (CTLs).

(a) These Tc CD8+ cells bind to the graft antigens via specific receptors and release **effector molecules**, such as perforins.

(b) **Perforins** create pores in the target cell membrane and enable serine proteases (i.e., granzymes) to enter the cell and initiate cell death by **apoptosis.**

(2) **Interferon-γ (IFN-γ)** activates monocytes/macrophages to express delayed-type hypersensitivity (DTH) toward transplant antigens. This reaction results in increased lysosomal activity, phagocytosis, respiratory burst, and the release of tumor necrosis factor-α (TNF-α).

(3) Activated **selectins, integrins, intercellular adhesion molecules (ICAM),** and **vascular cell adhesion molecules (VCAM)** promote **leukocyte extravasation** into the graft bed.

c. **Acute renal allograft rejection** results from injury to the renal vasculature by the Tc cells and their products, with resulting ischemia of the renal parenchyma.

d. **Second-set phenomenon** describes the rejection of a second allograft from the same donor as the initial allograft. The second allograft is rejected more quickly than the initial allograft (exhibiting the memory response).

2. **Chronic rejection**
   a. **Definition.** Chronic rejection is characterized by episodic bouts of rejection, occurring months to years after transplantation.
   b. **Mechanism of rejection.** Both cellular and humoral mechanisms are functional, eventually resulting in interstitial fibrosis, vascular occlusion, and loss of function.
3. **Hyperacute rejection**
   a. **Definition.** Hyperacute rejection occurs when a graft never takes because of preexisting sensitivity (white graft). **Rejection occurs within minutes.**
   b. **Mechanism of rejection.** The presence of **alloantibodies** against the donor's HLA or ABO antigens at the time of transplantation does not permit the graft to take. These antibodies react with the vascular endothelium of the graft and promote clotting, and thrombosis and necrosis cause rapid death of the organ.
   c. **Prevention. Cross-matching** donor and recipient cells and serum identifies this potential problem.

B. Graft-versus-host reaction
1. **Definition.** When **immunocompetent tissues** (e.g., bone marrow, thymus, spleen, organs harboring passenger leukocytes) are allografted, they may recognize the recipient (i.e., host) as foreign, resulting in CMI damage to the recipient. If the recipient is immunoincompetent, a host-versus-graft reaction does not take place.
2. **Signs and symptoms.** The reaction is characterized by a skin rash, diarrhea, and jaundice.
3. **Treatment.** Immunosuppressive therapy has proven useful in reducing lethality.

III **IMMUNOSUPPRESSION** is used to prolong graft acceptance; however, it predisposes the individual to infection.

A. Prevention of infection. Appropriate **killed (but no live) vaccines** should be administered before transplantation. **Major organisms that cause infection** include the following:
1. **Cytomegalovirus (CMV),** present in more than 50% of donors
2. ***Candida,*** present in more than 90% of donors
3. **Epstein-Barr virus,** present in more than 90% of donors
4. ***Aspergillus***
5. **Respiratory syncytial virus**

B. Immunosuppressive agents
1. **Cyclosporine A** is a metabolite of the fungus *Tolypocladium inflatum Gams.*
   a. **Mechanism of action.** Cyclosporine A **inhibits resting T cell activation** by blocking IL-2 mRNA synthesis. The drug **binds to a cyclophilin,** and then the cyclosporine–cyclophilin complex binds to **phosphatase calcineurin,** interfering with the transmission of intracellular signals necessary for IL-2 formation.
   b. Cyclosporine A has little effect on already activated cells; thus, **Rapamycin,** a macrolide isolated from *Streptomyces hygroscopicus* that binds to cyclophilins and inhibits the G1 phase of activated T cells, may be added.
2. **Tacrolimus (FK 506)** is a macrolide compound derived from *Streptomyces tsukabaensis* that also inhibits resting Th cell activation by blocking IL-2 synthesis. Tacrolimus binds to a different cyclophilin, FK-binding protein, and then the tacrolimus–cyclophilin complex inhibits calcineurin and IL-2 formation.
3. **Mycophenolate mofetil** inhibits inosine monophosphate dehydrogenase, an enzyme that converts inosine monophosphate to guanosine monophosphate. In

this way, mycophenolate mofetil **inhibits T and B cells**, because guanosine monophosphate is required for nucleic acid synthesis in these cells.

4. Other drugs

a. **Azathioprine**, a derivative of 6-mercaptopurine, is used early following transplantation. Azathioprine inhibits the synthesis of inosinic acid, thus blocking DNA synthesis in actively replicating cells.

b. **Corticosteroids** are anti-inflammatory agents that synergize with cyclosporine A.

(1) The corticosteroid bound receptor complexes with NF-κB to prevent transcription of IL-2 and other cytokines.

(2) Corticosteroids also suppress IL-2 synthesis indirectly by blocking macrophage release of IL-1.

c. **Antilymphocyte globulin (ALG)** is an antibody that causes lysis of recipient T lymphocytes reactive against the graft. ALG is most effective during acute rejection episodes.

Chapter 14

Cancer Immunology

DEFINITION. A **cancer** is a **malignant tumor growth** that expands locally by invasion and systemically by metastasis.

ONCOGENES. Cancers arise from cells in which growth-regulating and repair genes (**protooncogenes**) have become ineffective as a result of random mutation or following viral infection or physical or chemical damage. When protooncogenes become altered or damaged, they are termed **oncogenes** and are capable of causing neoplastic growth. Examples of oncogenes and their actions include the following.

A. **p53 gene.** As a protooncogene, p53 encodes a nuclear phosphoprotein that inhibits cell division, thus suppressing tumor growth. Mutations in p53 result in uncontrolled growth.

B. ***ras.*** As a protooncogene, *ras* controls a guanosine triphosphate (GTP) binding–protein involved in signal transduction. Mutation results in failure of guanosine triphosphatase (GTPase) inactivation of *ras* and continuous *ras* activity.

C. ***c-myc.*** When this protooncogene is translocated onto a different chromosome (e.g., as in Burkitt's lymphoma), it becomes oncogenic, resulting in loss of regulation of B cell growth and a B cell lymphoma.

D. **Bcl-2 gene.** In normal concentrations, the cellular protein produced by this gene (Bcl-2) inhibits apoptosis; high concentrations of Bcl-2 in B cells promote cell expansion and follicular lymphoma.

E. ***bcr/abl* gene fusion** results in a protein with increased tyrosine kinase activity and is involved in chronic myeloid leukemia.

CANCER AND THE IMMUNE SYSTEM

A. **Cancer antigens.** Cancer cells arise from normal cells. In order for the immune system to attack cancer cells, the **cancer cells** need to be distinguished from self (i.e., they **need to possess antigens**).

1. **Types.** Two types of antigenic molecules have been found on cancer cells.

   a. **Tumor-specific antigens (TSA)** are unique to cancer cells. They are induced by viruses (e.g., papovaviruses, herpesviruses, adenoviruses) or chemical or physical carcinogens.

      (1) **Virus-induced TSA** are **cross-reactive** (i.e., the genome of a particular virus synthesizes the same viral antigens in whatever cell that virus infects). Consequently, immunotherapy should be applicable to all individuals infected by the same virus.

      (2) **Carcinogen-induced TSA.** Carcinogens induce **random mutations** in the genome of affected cells. Consequently, each mutated gene product (antigen) differs (depending on which gene has been affected by the carcinogen), and immunologic cross-protection is not feasible.

b. **Tumor-associated antigens (TAA)** are not found exclusively on cancer cells; however, they are generally present in higher quantities in cancer patients and aid in diagnosis.
   (1) **Carcinoembryonic antigen (CEA)** reappears in the serum of most patients with colorectal cancer. (High concentrations of CEA on fetal gastrointestinal and liver cells normally disappear at birth.)
   (2) **β-Fetoprotein (AFP)** attains high levels in patients with hepatomas and testicular teratocarcinomas. Levels are normally very low in adults (although high AFP levels are normal in fetal and maternal serum).

2. **Immune response to cancer antigens**
   a. **Antigen-responsive T cells.** Immunocompromised hosts with diminished T cell function have a higher incidence of lymphoproliferative cancers.
      (1) **CD4+ T cells** secrete cytokines [e.g., interleukin-2 (IL-2), interferon-γ (IFN-γ)] that activate **CD8+ cytotoxic T cells (Tc)** and **macrophages.**
      (2) **CD8+ T cells** lyse cancer cells through cytotoxic factors and perforins.
   b. **Macrophages** are found frequently in the bed of regressing tumors. They must be activated by macrophage-activating factors (MAF), such as IFN-γ, in order to eradicate tumor cells. Mechanisms of destruction may include the respiratory burst, nitric oxide release, neutral proteinases, tumor necrosis factor-α (TNF-α), and antibody-dependent cell-mediated cytotoxicity (ADCC).
   c. **Natural killer (NK) cells** kill cancer cells through ADCC and lysis following contact. NK cell cytolytic activity is increased by IL-2, IL-12, and IFN-γ. Since they are not major histocompatibility complex (MHC) restricted, they can kill target cells that have low levels of MHC.

3. **Cancer cell evasion of the immune system.** Cancer cells can evade the immune system in multiple ways. Examples include the following:
   a. The relatively weak immune response may be overwhelmed by rapid tumor growth.
   b. Certain cancers may possess subliminal numbers of human leukocyte antigen (HLA) or costimultory signal molecules, rendering them unable to trigger a TSA T cell response.
   c. Non–complement fixing antibodies that arise as a result of the cancer may actually enhance cancer growth by blocking the TSA from attack by cell-mediated immunity (CMI).
   d. Certain cancers may elicit a dominant T cell suppressor (Ts) response or secrete immunosuppressive molecules [e.g., prostaglandins, transforming growth factor-β (TGF-β)].
   e. Antigenic modulation can occur, causing the cancer cells to change or lose their TSA.
   f. The cancer may arise in an immunologically privileged site [e.g., eye, central nervous system (CNS)].

IV CANCER IMMUNOTHERAPY

A. **Lymphokine-activated killer (LAK) cells** are tumor-reactive lymphocytes that are isolated from the blood of the cancer patient, expanded in vitro with IL-2, and reinfused into the patient. Although heterogenous, they are thought to constitute a population with some specificity. Their lineage is unknown, although most are NK cells.

B. **Tumor-infiltrating lymphocytes (TIL)** are T cells isolated from the tumor bed (therefore, they should have higher specificity for the tumor antigens). TIL cells are expanded in vitro with IL-2 and reinfused into the patient.

C. **Monoclonal antibodies** specific for TSA can be infused into the patient, either directly or with a toxin, drug, or radioisotope conjugated to the antibody. The antibody directs the conjugate exclusively to the cancer cell (e.g., humanized anti-CD20 for B cell lymphomas).

D. **Cytokine therapy**—using various cytokines capable of elevating humoral immunity, CMI, or both—is the goal of current clinical trials. The multiple variables (e.g., dose, concentration, bolus or multiple injections, route, patient population, cytokine specificity, toxicity) have impeded research progress.

Chapter 15

Immunization

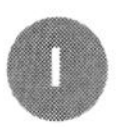

OVERVIEW

A. Benefits

1. Immunization is the most cost-effective weapon available against infectious diseases.
2. Immunization has permitted eradication of smallpox around the world and eradication of polio from the Western hemisphere. These successes are largely attributable to the Childhood Immunization Initiative passed by Congress in 1977.

B. Types of vaccines

1. **Live attenuated vaccines** permit replication of the organism (mainly viruses) in the host, increasing antigenic stimulation.
   a. Attenuation occurs mainly by passages in cell culture, growth in embryonic tissue or at low temperatures, or by selective deletion of genes involved in pathogenesis.
   b. A single inoculation frequently stimulates life-long immunity.
   c. Viral replication produces an MHC class I membrane display which activates CD8+ T cells.
2. **Killed vaccines** contain organisms that have been inactivated by chemical or physical means. Multiple doses must be given, and adjuvants might be required for a protective response.
3. **Recombinant vaccines** (e.g., hepatitis B vaccine). Formulation requires identification of an epitope involved in the organism's pathogenicity. Synthesis of the vaccine antigen follows isolation and expression of the gene coding for the epitope in an appropriate host cell.
4. **Plasmid DNA vaccines,** based on the isolation of microbial DNA containing the genes coding for an antigen involved in pathogenicity, are under development. Early results indicate that DNA vaccines elicit both potent humoral immunity and cell-mediated immunity (CMI) to multiple viruses and bacteria in animals; human clinical trials are in progress.
   a. **Advantages.** The potential advantages of DNA vaccines include stability, low cost, ease of production, and long-lasting protection.
   b. **Technique**
      (1) The DNA (gene) is inserted into an expression plasmid and transfected into bacteria, where the plasmid is replicated in large amounts. DNA from multiple pathogens can be inserted into a single large plasmid.
      (2) The isolated DNA can be either injected in saline solution or adsorbed to microscopic gold beads and fired into muscle cells with a "gene" gun.
      (3) The DNA is translated in the cells and the **antigen** of concern is released in vivo, stimulating humoral immunity and CMI over an extended period of time.

C. Requirements for an effective vaccine

1. **Protective effect.** The vaccine should induce a humoral or CMI response directed against an antigen involved in pathogenesis.
2. **Safety.** Potential safety problems must be recognized.
   a. **Live attenuated vaccines.** Potential safety problems include:
      (1) Insufficient attenuation
      (2) Reversion to wild type
      (3) Contamination by live organisms or toxins
      (4) Unsuspected immunodeficient patients
   b. **Killed vaccines.** Potential safety problems include:
      (1) Contamination by live organisms or toxins
      (2) Autoimmune or allergic reactions
      (3) Incomplete killing
   c. **Recombinant vaccines** are associated with few safety concerns.
   d. **Plasmid DNA vaccines.** Continuous antigenic stimulus may lead to tolerance or autoimmunity.
3. **Stability.** Most vaccines are stable for 1 year when maintained at a temperature of 4°C. They can deteriorate in 2–3 days at a temperature of 37°C.

II SPECIFIC VACCINES.

Current Minnesota vaccine recommendations are given in Table 15-1.

A. Hepatitis B vaccine. Hepatitis B virus, a hepadnavirus, is a major cause of hepatitis and cirrhosis and is a known human carcinogen.

1. **Vaccine production.** The vaccine antigen, **hepatitis B surface antigen (HBsAg)** appears on the surface membrane of the virus and in the blood of infected individuals. The noninfectious vaccine is produced by recombinant DNA technology.
   a. HBsAg is synthesized in *Saccharomyces cerevisiae* after the yeast is transfected with a plasmid containing the gene for HBsAg.
   b. The isolated and purified HBsAg protein is adsorbed onto aluminum hydroxide gel as adjuvant.
2. **Vaccine administration.** The hepatitis B vaccine is administered initially as an individual vaccine beginning before hospital discharge and during routine childhood vaccination, as indicated in Table 15.1.
3. **Postexposure prophylaxis. Hepatitis B immune globulin (HBIg)** is recommended for postexposure prophylaxis. Candidates include personnel in blood banks or transfusion units, pregnant women positive for circulating HBsAg, and newborns born to HBsAg-positive mothers.

B. Diphtheria and tetanus toxoids and acellular pertussis (DTaP) vaccine

1. **Vaccine production**
   a. **Diphtheria** and **tetanus** toxins are administered in the **toxoid form.**
   b. Pertussis is administered in the **acellular form,** which is associated with fewer adverse reactions than the whole-cell form.
2. **Vaccine administration.** The DTaP vaccine can be given at the same time as the trivalent oral polio vaccine (TOPV) and the measles-mumps-rubella (MMR) vaccine, but must be administered at a different site.

C. *Haemophilus influenzae* type b (Hib) vaccine. *H. influenzae* type b was the major cause of bacterial meningitis in the United States prior to licensure of the Hib conjugate vaccines.

1. **Vaccine production.** The Hib vaccine incorporates the polysaccharide antigen, a polymer of polyribosyl ribitolphosphate (PRP) found in the type b capsule (the major virulence component in 90% of the invasive strains). PRP, a thymus-

TABLE 15.1 RECOMMENDED CHILDHOOD AND ADOLESCENT IMMUNIZATION SCHEDULE, MINNESOTA, 2004
****Chart must be used with guidelines below****

Range of recommended ages				Catch-up vaccination				Preadolescent assessment			
Vaccine / **Age**	Birth	1 mo	2 mos	4 mos	6 mos	12 mos	15 mos	18 mos	24 mos	4-6 yrs	11-12 yrs	13-18 yrs
Hepatitis B[1]	HepB-1	only if mother is HBsAg(-)	HepB-2			HepB-3					HepB series	
Diphtheria, Tetanus, Pertussis[2]			DTaP	DTaP	DTaP			DTaP[2]		DTaP	Td[2]	
***Haemophilus influenzae* type b[3]**			Hib	Hib	Hib[3]	Hib[3]						
Inactivated Poliovirus			IPV	IPV		IPV				IPV		
Measles, Mumps, Rubella[4]						MMR-1				MMR-2[4]	MMR-2[4]	
Varicella[5]							Varicella				Varicella	
Pneumococcal[6]			PCV	PCV	PCV	PCV			PCV	PPV		
Vaccine below this line is for selected populations												
Influenza[7]						Influenza (yearly) *as of fall 2004*					Influenza (yearly)	
Hepatitis A[8]											HepA series	

Guidelines: This schedule is for children through age 18 yrs. It indicates the recommended ages for routine administration of childhood vaccines licensed as of January 1, 2004. Any dose not given at the recommended age should be given at any subsequent visit when indicated and feasible. [shaded box] Indicates age groups that warrant special effort to administer those vaccines not previously given. Additional vaccines may be licensed and recommended during the year. Licensed combination vaccines may be used whenever any components of the combination are indicated and the vaccine's other components are not contraindicated. Consult the manufacturers' package inserts for detailed recommendations.

independent antigen, can be conjugated to protein carriers [e.g., diphtheria toxoid, *Neisseria meningitidis* outer membrane protein (OMP), tetanus toxoid], rendering it highly protective in children older than 2 months.

2. **Vaccine administration.** PRP-OMP and PRP-tetanus toxoid are given in 3–4 doses, beginning at the age of 2 months; PRP-diphtheria toxoid is recommended only for children older than 1 year.

D. **Poliomyelitis vaccines.** Poliomyelitis is caused by three serotypes of poliovirus; type 1 causes paralytic disease most often.

1. **Available vaccines.** Two vaccines are available.
   a. **Trivalent oral polio vaccine (TOPV)** contains **live attenuated** strains of all three serotypes of poliovirus, which are propagated in monkey kidney cell cultures.
      (1) TOPV is administered **orally.**
      (2) TOPV induces **local** and **systemic immunity**—local immunity is accomplished by proliferation of the virus in the gastrointestinal tract, and systemic immunity is accomplished by spread of the attenuated virus to the circulation.
   b. **Inactivated polio vaccine (IPV)** contains **killed virus.**
      (1) IPV is administered **subcutaneously.**
      (2) IPV induces a **systemic** immune response.
2. **Vaccination schedule**
   a. A schedule of two doses of IPV followed by two doses of TOPV decreases the risk of vaccine-associated poliomyelitis. The initial antibody response induced by the IPV protects the patient against the remote possibility that vaccine-associated disease might be caused by the subsequent TOPV.
   b. TOPV-only and IPV-only regimens are also acceptable for human use.

E. **Measles-mumps-rubella (MMR) vaccine.** This vaccine has decreased the incidence of measles, mumps, and rubella by 99%. In addition, the MMR vaccine has decreased the incidence of major birth defects (associated with rubella), encephalitis (associated with measles), and aseptic meningitis and parotitis (associated with mumps).

1. **Vaccine production**
   a. **Measles** and **mumps**, paramyxoviruses, are grown in chick embryo cell cultures.
   b. **Rubella**, a togavirus, is grown in human diploid fibroblast cell cultures.
2. **Vaccine administration**
   a. Two doses are required prior to school enrollment.
   b. MMR, a live vaccine, should not be administered to pregnant women.
   c. The vaccine is heat- and light-sensitive.

F. **Varicella vaccine.** Varicella-zoster virus causes chickenpox.

1. **Vaccine production.** The vaccine is formulated from a **live attenuated virus.**
2. **Vaccine administration.** Vaccination is recommended for children between the ages of 1 and 12 years and for adults who have not contracted chickenpox.

G. **Hepatitis A vaccine**

1. **Vaccine production.** Hepatitis A, a picornavirus (enterovirus), is grown in cultures of human fibroblasts. The purified virus is inactivated by formalin and adsorbed onto an aluminum hydroxide gel to make the vaccine.
2. **Vaccine indications.** People in close contact with patients with hepatitis A, people with high occupational risk, homosexuals, and travelers should be vaccinated.
3. **Postexposure prophylaxis** with **anti-hepatitis A immunoglobulin** is warranted.

H. Influenza virus vaccine

1. **Classification of influenza virus.** The classification of influenza virus into types A, B, and C is based on differences in the nucleoproteins.
2. **Vaccine production**
    a. Influenza type A virus has two important surface antigens, a **hemagglutinin (H)** and a **neuraminidase (N)**; variations in each determine the subtypes of the type A influenza virus.
        (1) Three subtypes of hemagglutinins are recognized (H1, H2, H3). **Antibody to the hemagglutinins reduces the likelihood of infection and lessens the severity of disease.**
        (2) Two subtypes of neuraminidase (N1 and N2) exist.
    b. The vaccine is an **attenuated virus vaccine** that **contains three virus strains**, usually **two type A strains** and **one type B strain.** (Type C is not an important human pathogen.)
        (1) The strains chosen each year represent the influenza viruses that are most likely to circulate in the United States during the upcoming influenza season.
        (2) **Antigenic drift** results from mutations in the RNA segment coding for either of the major membrane antigens. Type A strains exhibit much greater antigenic variation than type B strains. No cross-protection between strains occurs.
    c. The vaccine is made from highly purified, egg-grown viruses that have been inactivated. Whole virus, subvirion, and purified surface antigen preparations are available.
3. **Vaccine indications.** The vaccine is indicated for most patients, especially those older than 65 years and residents of nursing homes or other chronic care facilities.
4. **Vaccine administration**
    a. **Subvirion** or **purified surface antigen vaccines** cause fewer febrile reactions, and are used in **patients younger than 12 years.**
    b. The vaccine should be **withheld from patients with known anaphylactic hypersensitivity to eggs.**
5. **Influenza vaccine composition.** Influenza vaccines are named according to the following sequence: virus type, geographic origin, strain number, year of isolation, and the type A virus subtype. Both the inactivated and live, attenuated vaccines prepared for the 2004–2005 season included A/Fujian/411/2002 (H3N2)-like, A/New Caledonia/20/99 (H1N1)-like, and B/Shanghai/361/2002-like antigens. For the A/Fujian/411/2002 (H3N2)-like antigen, manufacturers may use the antigenically equivalent A/Wyoming/3/2003 (H3N2) virus, and for the B/Shanghai/361/2002-like antigen, manufacturers may use the antigenically equivalent B/Jilin/20/2003 virus or B/Jiangsu/10/2003 virus. These viruses are used because of their growth properties and because they are representative of influenza viruses likely to circulate in the United States during the 2004–2005 influenza season. Because circulating influenza A (H1N2) viruses are a reassortant of influenza A (H1N1) and (H3N2) viruses, antibody directed against influenza A (H1N1) and influenza (H3N2) vaccine strains will provide protection against circulating influenza A (H1N2) viruses. Influenza viruses for both the inactivated and live attenuated influenza vaccines are initially grown in embryonated hens' eggs. Thus, both vaccines might contain limited amounts of residual egg protein. (Taken from: Recommendations of the Advisory Committee on Immunization Practices (ACIP), MMWR 2004;53[RR06]:1–40.)

I. *Streptococcus pneumoniae* vaccine. The capsule is the primary pathogenic element of the pneumococcus. Anticapsular antibody, which appears after a 2- to 3-week induction period, is completely protective, increasing opsonization, phagocytosis, and killing of the bacteria.

1. **Vaccine production.** The *S. pneumoniae* vaccine is composed of **23 polysaccharides** purified from the capsules of the most important serotypes.
   a. The polysaccharides are **thymus-independent antigens**, which are not effective in children younger than 2 years. Complexing the antigens with carrier proteins or absorbing them into liposomes can convert them to a thymus-dependent state.
   b. Little or no memory is produced; however, the polysaccharides persist in tissues and continue to stimulate antibody synthesis.
2. **Vaccine administration.** The antibody response persists for approximately 5 years, at which time revaccination is recommended for asplenic patients, those with chronic illnesses, and those older than 65 years. Revaccination is not recommended if the individual was vaccinated initially after the age of 65.

J. A new pediatric *combination* vaccine (Pediarix) was approved in 2002. It protects infants against diphtheria, tetanus, whooping cough, polio and hepatitis B virus.

1. It contains DTaP (diphtheria and tetanus toxoids and acellular pertussis vaccine, adsorbed), hepatitis B vaccine (recombinant), and inactivated poliovirus vaccine.
2. The individual vaccines are given together as a single injection intramuscularly three times at 2, 4, and 6 months of age, thus reducing the number of injections from ~9 to 3.

III

ADJUVANTS are substances that can be added to vaccines to increase their immunogenicity.

A. Aluminum hydroxide gel is the only adjuvant for vaccines currently approved for human use.

1. The antigen is adsorbed onto the gel when aluminum chloride is treated with sodium hydroxide.
2. The antigen is released slowly and large numbers of antigen-presenting cells (APCs) are attracted to the injection site, increasing and prolonging antibody formation.
3. The adsorbed antigen exhibits minimal toxicity; occasionally, granulomas form at the site of injection.

B. Other compounds with diverse capabilities for enhancing any of the many steps leading to humoral immunity and CMI are under study for inclusion in human vaccine preparations, including **cytokines, chemokines,** and **synthetic bacteria-derived lipids.**

Study Questions and Answers

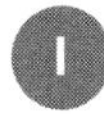

Comprehensive Review Questions

1. Specific receptors binding antigens appear on T lymphocytes
   - **A.** following contact with antigens in the fetal thymus
   - **B.** following contact with antigens in peripheral lymphoid organs
   - **C.** only after contact with antigens processed by APC
   - **D.** independent of antigen contact

2. The major antigenic receptor on a B cell membrane
   - **A.** is the same structurally as the antigen receptor on a T cell
   - **B.** is a monomeric IgM molecule
   - **C.** is a pentameric IgM molecule
   - **D.** is a monomeric IgG molecule

3. The epitope specificity of a particular B cell clone
   - **A.** is determined by interaction with antigen
   - **B.** is determined by the kappa chain sequence
   - **C.** is determined by the mu chain constant region
   - **D.** is determined by both the H and L chain hypervariable regions
   - **E.** changes after isotype switching

4. The antigenic determinants defining the 5 IG isotypes are associated with
   - **A.** kappa light chains
   - **B.** lambda light chains
   - **C.** heavy chains
   - **D.** J chains
   - **E.** di-sulphide bonds

5. Antiserum developed in rabbits against pooled human IgA will react with human
   - **A.** kappa light chains
   - **B.** IgM
   - **C.** IgG
   - **D.** J chain
   - **E.** each of the above

6. Phagocytosis of a microbe involves
   - **A.** endocytosis of the microbe in a phagocytic vacuole
   - **B.** merging of the phagocytic vacuole with a lysosome particle
   - **C.** disruption of the microbe by lysosomal enzymes

D. attachment of the antigenic fragments to HLA molecules
E. each of the above events is correct
F. none of the above statements is correct

7. The secretory piece
A. facilitates passage of IgA out of the plasma cell
B. facilitates the formation of the IgM pentamer
C. joins the two molecules of IgA forming the dimmer
D. is a poly Ig receptor on the membranes of mucosal epithelial cells
E. is released by IgE, causing excessive nasal secretions

8. Which of the following statements is INCORRECT?
A. T cells bearing the alpha/beta receptor give rise to both CD4+ and CD8+ cells.
B. CD4+ cells give rise to both Th1 and Th2+ cells.
C. Th1 cells secrete IL-2.
D. Th2 cells secrete IL-4.
E. Th2 cells increase cell-mediated immunity.

9. The immunoglobulin that has four subclasses is
A. IgM
B. IgG
C. IgA
D. IgE
E. IgD

10. A hapten
A. stimulates T cell responses
B. stimulates B cell responses
C. enhances the antibody response by forming a depot for the antigen
D. activates macrophages for increased phagocytosis
E. requires a carrier to initiate an immune response

11. A super-antigen
A. attaches to the epitope binding region of the HLA molecule
B. binds to both T and B cells
C. attaches to the IgM receptor on B cells
D. causes the secretion of abnormally high concentrations of cytokines
E. binds to both the IgM and IgD receptors on B cells

12. Class II HLA molecules
A. present peptidic epitopes to CD4+ T helper cells
B. present peptidic epitopes to CD8+ T helper cells
C. are encoded by the gene regions DP, DQ, DR
D. appear on the membranes of most nucleated cells
E. are characterized by each of the above

13. Pepsin digestion of an IgG antibody against tetanus toxoid will
A. result in loss of the ability to form a lattice with the toxoid
B. produce two Fab molecules and one Fc fragment
C. produce a (Fab)2 molecule and loss of the ability of the Fc fragment to bind to macrophages

D. loss of the L chains
E. loss of the C1 heavy chain constant domain

14. The cluster of differentiation (CD) functional as a co-receptor on T cells that exhibit cell-mediated immunity is
A. CD2
B. CD3
C. CD4
D. CD8

15. Thymus independent antigens
A. are usually multiple-branched polysaccharides
B. are usually high-molecular-weight proteins
C. are MHC restricted
D. are usually mucoproteins

16. The Fc fragment of an IgG antibody
A. can attach to a receptor on macrophages
B. permits passage through the placenta
C. can participate in the activation of complement
D. determines the catabolic rate of IgG
E. is characterized by each of the above

17. The T cell antigenic receptor
A. is a monomeric IgM molecule
B. is a monomeric IgG molecule
C. will respond only to epitopes processed by class I HLA molecules
D. does not interact directly with circulating antigens

18. HLA molecules
A. discriminate between self and non-self
B. present processed antigen to T cells of the same HLA types
C. are highly polymorphic
D. control susceptibility to certain immunologic disorders
E. are characterized by each of the above

19. The most important Ig protecting a 1-month-old baby is
A. IgM
B. IgG
C. IgA
D. IgE
E. IgD

20. Which of these statements is INCORRECT?
A. Most fetal thymocytes die in apoptosis.
B. Apoptosis is characterized by membrane blebbing and DNA fragmentation.
C. The alpha/beta T cell receptor responds to peptide antigens bound to HLA molecules.
D. Th2 cell cytokines induce B cell transformation and proliferation.
E. Th1 cells secrete IL-4, IL-5, and IL-6 cytokines.

21. The Ig with the longest serum half-life is designated
- **A.** alpha 2, kappa 2
- **B.** delta 2, kappa 2
- **C.** epsilon 2, kappa 2
- **D.** gamma 2, kappa 2
- **E.** mu 2, kappa 2

22. On entry into a lymph node, viral antigens
- **A.** are synthesized endogenously within the antigen presenting cell
- **B.** are synthesized endogenously within the T lymphocyte
- **C.** are synthesized endogenously within the B lymphocyte
- **D.** bind to the MHC class I complex without being broken down

23. Interferon-gamma can
- **A.** trigger HLA antigen presentation by endothelial cells
- **B.** activate macrophages
- **C.** down-regulate interleukin-4 synthesis
- **D.** do each of the above
- **E.** do none of the above

24. Which of the following stimulates the acute phase response?
- **A.** Interferon-gamma
- **B.** Interleukin-2
- **C.** Interleukin-5
- **D.** Tumor necrosis factor-alpha
- **E.** Perforin

25. Which interleukin is necessary for the switch to IgE production?
- **A.** 1
- **B.** 2
- **C.** 4
- **D.** 5
- **E.** 6

26. Activation of T helper cells by antigen-presenting cells requires
- **A.** CD2
- **B.** CD3
- **C.** CD4
- **D.** CD28
- **E.** each of the above is required

27. Which of the following statements is INCORRECT?
- **A.** T cytotoxic cells have the CD8+ phenotype
- **B.** Interleukin-8 is a chemotactic agent for neutrophils
- **C.** Interleukin-1 and TNF-alpha induce selectins on the endothelial cell surface
- **D.** Interleukin-4, IL-10, and TGF-beta are the main cause of excessive inflammation
- **E.** NK cells can express antibody-dependent cellular cytotoxicity

28. Which of the following is an example of type II hypersensitivity?
- **A.** Goodpasture's glomerulonephritis
- **B.** Serum sickness
- **C.** Post-streptococcal nephritis

D. Arthus reaction
E. Asthma

29. Differentiation of antibody classes is a property of
A. V_L chain region
B. V_H chain region
C. C_L chain region
D. C_H chain region
E. hinge region

30. With respect to genetic control of heavy chain synthesis
A. the variable region is coded by three different gene complexes
B. a J region gene links first to a D region gene and then to a V region gene
C. a VDJ complex links to a mu region gene
D. each of the above occurs

31. Which statement is INCORRECT?
A. Class I HLA molecules are found on most nucleated cells.
B. Class II HLA molecules are found on immunocompetent cells.
C. Class I HLA molecules are linked to T cells via the CD8 molecule.
D. Class II HLA molecules are linked to T cells via the CD4 molecule.
E. Class II has three gene regions labeled A, B, and C.

32. Which statement is INCORRECT?
A. IL-1 induces acute phase reactants.
B. IL-2 is a growth factor for Th2 cells.
C. IL-4 inhibits IgE synthesis.
D. TGF-beta is an immunosuppressant.
E. IL-8 induces neutrophil chemotaxis.

33. Which statement is INCORRECT?
A. Cross-linkage by antigen of two or more IgE molecules is required for degranulation of sensitized mast cells.
B. Damage during type II reactions can be caused by either opsonization or complement lysis.
C. dsDNA-anti-dsDNA complexes can initiate glomerulonephritis.
D. Contact dermatitis due to poison ivy is an Ag-Ab complex lesion.
E. Macrophages are activated non-specifically by interferon-gamma.

34. Which of these serum values (mgm %) would indicate an immunodeficiency disease?
A. IgA $\rightarrow$ 100–300
B. IgG $\rightarrow$ 200–400
C. IgM $\rightarrow$ 60–200
D. Each of the above

35. Which of these statements concerning AIDS is INCORRECT?
A. Both CD4+ T cells and macrophages can be infected.
B. HIV requires both CD4 and a chemokine co-receptor to enter cells.
C. HIV reverse transcriptase changes viral RNA into DNA.
D. Latent provirus formation follows integration of viral DNA into the host genome by an integrase.
E. CD4+ T cell levels at 1200/μL predispose to cytomegalous virus infection.

36. A fundamental characteristic of innate immunity is
- **A.** adaptable responses toward many different antigens
- **B.** rapid recognition and response to pathogens
- **C.** expression of antigen receptors
- **D.** long-term immunity with memory

37. The role of natural killer cells is
- **A.** to recognize cells expressing MHC class II molecules
- **B.** to recognize cells expressing MHC class I molecules
- **C.** to recognize cells with deficient expression of MHC class II molecules
- **D.** to recognize cells with deficient expression of MHC class I molecules
- **E.** to recognize tumor and viral antigens

38. The function of mature dendritic cells is
- **A.** to capture bacteria
- **B.** to present antigen
- **C.** to migrate in tissues looking for pathogenic antigens
- **D.** to produce IL-2
- **E.** to direct inflammatory responses

39. Innate immune cells mount cell-mediated immune responses to specific antigens by
- **A.** recognition with α:β receptors
- **B.** recognition with δ:γ receptors
- **C.** recognition with surface monomeric IgM
- **D.** recognition with toll-like receptors
- **E.** recognition with antigen-specific immunoglobulin bound by Fc receptors

40. Activation of Janus kinases requires
- **A.** recruitment of STAT to the receptor
- **B.** cytokine binding to the receptor
- **C.** oligomerization of the cytokine receptor
- **D.** receptor phosphorylation
- **E.** receptor complexes with an Src kinase

41. Src kinase activity is activated by
- **A.** recruitment to a receptor
- **B.** phosphorylation of a tyrosine group in the active site
- **C.** phosphorylation of ITAM groups
- **D.** phosphorylation by Csk to cause a protein folding event
- **E.** de-phosphorylation of a regulatory tyrosine phosphate in the active site

42. Scaffolding is assembled by
- **A.** attaching protein modules using SH3 groups
- **B.** attaching phosphoserine groups to SH2 groups
- **C.** attaching phosphotyrosine groups to SH2 groups
- **D.** attaching between conserved immunoglobulin folds
- **E.** recruiting multiple receptors

43. An important function of the T cell receptor is
- **A.** initiating signal transduction
- **B.** regulating the activation of CD8 versus CD4 cells

C. recognizing antigen
D. recognizing antigen-MHC complexes
E. recruit mDC2

44. Which of the following is an example of type III hypersensitivity?
A. asthma
B. systemic lupus erythematosus
C. myasthenia gravis
D. rhinitis
E. contact dermatitis

45. Immediate hypersensitivity skin reactions
A. exhibit a wheal due to influx of mononuclear cells
B. exhibit a red flare due to vasodilation
C. cannot be elicited by monovalent haptens
D. are due to IgE antibody
E. all of the above are correct

46. Which of the following diseases involves a reaction to a hapten?
A. Goodpasture's syndrome
B. Rheumatoid arthritis
C. Arthus reaction
D. Anaphylaxis following penicillin treatment
E. Each of the above diseases

47. Serum sickness occurs only when
A. anti-basement membrane antibodies are present
B. extreme excess of antibody is present
C. IgE antibody is produced
D. soluble immune complexes are formed
E. neutrophils are absent

48. A major marker retained on all peripheral T cells is
A. CD3
B. CD4
C. CD8
D. IL-1
E. IL-2

49. CD34 is a marker for
A. Th1 cells
B. Th2 cells
C. Gamma-delta T cell receptor
D. B cells
E. Stem cells

50. Which statement is INCORRECT?
A. A hapten can bind an epitope.
B. A superantigen binds to the peptide-binding site of many alpha-beta T cell receptors.
C. Thymus independent antigens can activate B cells.
D. Thymus independent antigens are mainly multi-branched polysaccharides.

51. Tolerance to self antigens can be achieved by
- **A.** clonal deletion
- **B.** clonal anergy
- **C.** high doses of antigen
- **D.** low doses of antigen
- **E.** each of the above

52. Congenital agammaglobulinemia (Brutons disease) would most likely exhibit the characteristic(s):
- **A.** a genetic defect in the NADPH oxidase system
- **B.** a loss in the enzyme adenosine deaminase
- **C.** a triad of thrombocytopenia, eczema, and recurrent infections
- **D.** an absence of T cells, hypocalcemia, and tetany
- **E.** requires the chemokine CCR-5 for the disease to progress
- **F.** a defect in the transition from pre-B cells to B cells
- **G.** a selective loss in IgA levels

53. Characteristics of multiple sclerosis would likely include
- **A.** an anti-acetylcholine antibody
- **B.** an anti–anti-acetylcholine receptor antibody
- **C.** increased CNS fluid antibody titers to viruses
- **D.** an increase in suppressor T cell functions
- **E.** each of the above

54. Dysgammaglobulinemia would most likely exhibit the characteristic(s):
- **A.** a genetic defect in the NADPH oxidase system
- **B.** a loss in the enzyme adenosine deaminase
- **C.** a triad of thrombocytopenia, eczema, and recurrent infections
- **D.** an absence of T cells, hypocalcemia, and tetany
- **E.** requires the chemokine CCR-5 for the disease to progress
- **F.** a defect in the transition from pre-B cells to B cells
- **G.** a selective loss in IgA levels

55. Congenital thymic aplasia (DiGeorge syndrome) is most likely to exhibit the characteristic(s):
- **A.** a genetic defect in the NADPH oxidase system
- **B.** a loss in the enzyme adenosine deaminase
- **C.** a triad of thrombocytopenia, eczema, and recurrent infections
- **D.** an absence of T cells, hypocalcemia, and tetany
- **E.** requires the chemokine CCR-5 for the disease to progress
- **F.** a defect in the transition from pre-B cells to B cells
- **G.** a selective loss in IgA levels

56. Wiskott-Aldrich syndrome is most likely to exhibit the characteristic(s):
- **A.** a genetic defect in the NADPH oxidase system
- **B.** a loss in the enzyme adenosine deaminase
- **C.** a triad of thrombocytopenia, eczema, and recurrent infections
- **D.** an absence of T cells, hypocalcemia, and tetany
- **E.** requires the chemokine CCR-5 for the disease to progress
- **F.** a defect in the transition from pre-B cells to B cells
- **G.** a selective loss in IgA levels

57. Pernicious anemia patients are characterized by:
A. antibodies against the parietal cell
B. antibodies against intrinsic factor
C. T cell damage to the gastric parietal cell
D. inhibition of vitamin B_{12} transport
E. each of the above

58. Severe combined immunodeficiency disease is most likely to exhibit the characteristic(s):
A. a genetic defect in the NADPH oxidase system
B. a loss in the enzyme adenosine deaminase
C. a triad of thrombocytopenia, eczema, and recurrent infections
D. an absence of T cells, hypocalcemia, and tetany
E. requires the chemokine CCR-5 for the disease to progress
F. a defect in the transition from pre-B cells to B cells
G. a selective loss in IgA levels

59. Chronic granulomatous disease is most likely to exhibit the characteristic(s):
A. a genetic defect in the NADPH oxidase system
B. a loss in the enzyme adenosine deaminase
C. a triad of thrombocytopenia, eczema, and recurrent infections
D. an absence of T cells, hypocalcemia, and tetany
E. requires the chemokine CCR-5 for the disease to progress
F. a defect in the transition from pre-B cells to B cells
G. a selective loss in IgA levels

60. Ulcerative colitis is characterized by:
A. an inflammatory lesion confined to the rectum and colon
B. infiltration of monocytes, lymphocytes, and plasma cells
C. lymphocyte cytotoxicity against cultured colonic epithelial cells
D. antibodies reacting with *Escherichia coli*
E. each of the above

61. Acquired immunodeficiency disease syndrome is most likely to exhibit the characteristic(s):
A. a genetic defect in the NADPH oxidase system
B. a loss in the enzyme adenosine deaminase
C. a triad of thrombocytopenia, eczema, and recurrent infections
D. an absence of T cells, hypocalcemia, and tetany
E. requires the chemokine CCR-5 for the disease to progress
F. a defect in the transition from pre-B cells to B cells
G. a selective loss in IgA levels

62. Graves disease is characterized by:
A. antibodies to the thyroid stimulating hormone
B. antibodies to the thyroid stimulating hormone receptor
C. antibodies to thyroid peroxidase
D. hypothyroidism
E. each of the above

63. Which of these viral vaccines has as its major antigens a hemagglutinin and a neuraminidase?
A. Oral polio vaccine
B. Measles-mumps-rubella

C. Influenza type A
D. Hepatitis A
E. Hepatitis B

64. Which of the following statements is INCORRECT?
A. The diphtheria-tetanus-acellular pertussis vaccine can be given at the same time as measles-mumps-rubella vaccine.
B. The trivalent oral polio vaccine can proliferate in the gastrointestinal tract.
C. The hepatitis B vaccine is given during the first month of life.
D. The *Streptococcus pneumoniae* vaccine does not give a secondary memory response.

65. Which immunosuppressive agent inhibits resting T cell activation by blocking IL-2 mRNA synthesis?
A. Cyclosporin A
B. Mycophenolate mofetil
C. Azathioprine
D. Corticosteroid
E. Anti-lymphocyte globulin

66. Which statement with respect to organ transplantation is INCORRECT?
A. A graft versus host reaction does not occur with a thymus graft.
B. A graft versus host reaction does not occur in an immunoincompetent recipient
C. A xenograft is between members of a different species
D. Class I HLA antigens are found on all nucleated cells
E. Class II HLA antigens are found on immunologic effector cells

67. Which protooncogene encodes a nuclear phosphatase that when mutated causes uncontrolled cell division?
A. *ras*
B. p53
C. *c-myc*
D. Bcl-2

Answers

QUESTION NUMBER	ANSWER	QUESTION NUMBER	ANSWER
1.	D	35.	E
2.	B	36.	B
3.	D	37.	D
4.	C	38.	B
5.	E	39.	E
6.	E	40.	C
7.	D	41.	B
8.	E	42.	C
9.	B	43.	D
10.	E	44.	B
11.	D	45.	E
12.	A	46.	D
13.	C	47.	D
14.	D	48.	A
15.	A	49.	E
16.	E	50.	B
17.	D	51.	E
18.	E	52.	F
19.	B	53.	C
20.	E	54.	G
21.	D	55.	D
22.	A	56.	C
23.	D	57.	E
24.	D	58.	B
25.	C	59.	A
26.	E	60.	E
27.	D	61.	E
28.	A	62.	B
29.	D	63.	C
30.	D	64.	A
31.	E	65.	A
32.	C	66.	A
33.	D	67.	B
34.	B